TREATING PROBLEMS NOT SYMPTOMS

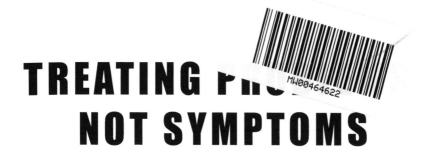

Your Official Guide to Keeping Active, Maintaining Your Independence, and Living Without Pain Medications... Into Your 60s, 70s, 80s, and Beyond!

by Florida's leading physical therapist
Dr. Jake Berman, PT, DPT

Publisher: Dr. Jake Berman, 501 Goodlette Rd. N. Ste. C-100, Naples, FL 34102

While they have made every effort to verify the information here, neither the author nor the publisher assumes any responsibility for errors in, omissions from, or a different interpretation of the subject matter. This information may be subject to varying laws and practices in different areas, states, and countries.

The reader assumes all responsibility for the use of the information.

The author and publisher shall in no event be held liable to any party for any damages arising directly or indirectly from any use of this material. Every effort has been made to accurately represent this product and its potential.

Printed in the United States of America.

ISBN 9781728650869

CONTENTS

Testimonials
Acknowledgements
About the Author

PART I: A PARADIGM SHIFT

Testimonials

My husband Don had a stroke. He was having so much difficulty even getting out of a chair. We went for a consultation at Berman Physical Therapy, and the moment we went in the door, we knew it was definitely the right place. The compassion and concern for getting my husband up out of the chair and walking again was amazing! Our therapist's techniques and knowledge for what was going on with my husband was remarkable. I'm happy to say my husband is doing so well and is out walking as I write. **We've been to many therapists but NONE can compare to what Berman Physical Therapy has accomplished with my husband.**

—Donna, 70

Absolutely outstanding. I fell in June, had a knee replacement in September, and came down to Naples in January. That whole time I was in miserable pain. I saw three PT's, two chiropractors and an orthopedic. Nothing worked. **Berman Physical Therapy fixed me.** It's that simple.

—Fred, 63

The staff at BPT are the best. After a severe broken leg, my recovery stalled and reversed to the point that my daughters thought I would be crippled for life. Then I was referred to Berman PT when I arrived in Naples for the winter. **From day one, I received relief from my pain and numbness and put on a progressive exercise program that put me on a path to recovery.** They also found a comparable PT practice to continue my therapy when I returned to Boston in March. I highly recommend BPT without reservation and I very much appreciate the caring and effective treatment that I received there.

—Cathy, 68

Everyone at Berman Physical Therapy is extremely knowledgeable about human physiology and pain management. **Their techniques are very different from other physical therapists, at least the ones that I've seen over the years (and I've seen my fair share).** They also are far more effective in identifying and correcting muscular or skeletal issues that cause chronic pain. I would highly recommend them without any reservation or qualification. They are not inexpensive, but if you do what they tell you to do, you will get your money's worth…and then some.

—*Dr. Robert, 71*

Best decision I ever made was to make an appointment at Berman Physical Therapy. I had a referral from a friend and I read through some positive google reviews before I called the office to ask a few questions and spoke to Elizabeth. I immediately felt confident with the office and booked a free consultation with Dr David Lee to discuss my neck and back issues. I was very impressed with Dr David and booked my first treatment right away. The treatment has had an extremely positive impact.

—*David, 33*

I had lower back pain daily for almost one year. **After spending time with David at Berman PT I can say my daily pain is 95% gone.** I have learned so much and now feel control of pain symptoms is under my control. I believe if you do the work you can regain a heathy back. Thanks so much for being there.

—*Pete, 75*

I hadn't been able to swing a golf club in four months. I went to Berman PT twice a week for five weeks, and then I was back to playing golf again. I had seen two other doctors before this with no help. **I can't say enough about Berman Physical Therapy.**

—*Doc, 66*

From the minute you walk into Berman Physical Therapy you are greeted with a positive, warm and supportive staff! I have seen many therapists for my condition. No one, in my experience, has worked harder to find out exactly what will help my recovery. **You will get your money's worth and more.**

—Ellen, 56

I always leave feeling better than when I came in. Berman PT is not your typical physical therapy office. The doctors are very confident and knowledgeable and provide the best Manual Therapy. They re-evaluates and makes changes each visit based on your progress and abilities. They will also provide you with a well-thought-out home program to encourage further healing.

—Kella, 64

I came to Berman Physical Therapy with plantar fasciitis in my right foot and a soft tissue injury in my left leg which recently had a hip replaced. I was in a lot of pain and struggled to walk. A PT in my home state aggravated my condition, so I came in skeptical of a good result. Well, I got one. By my 2nd visit the plantar fasciitis was 90% gone. **The Berman PT staff knows what they are doing and I wouldn't go to anyone else.**

—Charlene, 61

Always a pleasant experience at Berman Physical Therapy. The whole team is very attentive, knowledgeable, and caring. **Their therapists give me complete attention and always go the extra mile to explain my injuries in terms that I can understand,** along with taking time to listen to all symptoms and answering any questions I have. They keep a welcoming atmosphere and make sure I leave with all the knowledge needed to continue on the positive track to recovery.

—Mike, 32

I have been to a number of other P.T.s in the past with mixed results. **Berman Physical Therapy's approach to care is markedly different.** They are completely hands-on, which keeps them focused on the goals you have set together during the initial workup. They are constantly thinking and adapting their techniques so that when something doesn't work they can make corrections and adapt their approach to get results.

—Dr. Ted, 70

I would be happy to recommend Berman Physical Therapy to others. I have been appreciative of their help, which has been more than meaningful. **I think they are focused on the best straight line to fix the problem and do a very good job communicating the how and why of what needs to be done.** They are also obviously knowledgeable and engaged. They do a great job.

—John, 72

I had right hip pain that bothered me for probably three years. I had tried other therapies with no permanent relief. I came to Berman Physical Therapy and within 6 weeks with a combination of office visits and "homework," I was pain-free. They have also helped me with shoulder/scapula pain which, is greatly improved. **These guys know their stuff!!** Everyone in the office is just plain fun!

—Denise, 69

I have been to a lot of PTs in my life and Berman Physical Therapy is unique. Their approach is holistic, yet pragmatic. I had back surgery a few years ago and when I went to Berman PT the reason for the surgery was starting to come back. It's gone now. **They used a combination of hands-on therapy and exercises that really worked**—and everyone there is smart, amusing, and nice.

—Penny, 63

This was my first time working with a Dr. of Physical Therapy, and I was pleasantly surprised. My therapist at Berman PT identified the cause of my pain and immediately went to work—with immediate results. **Their commitment to patient education was both welcome and refreshing.** I highly recommend Berman Physical Therapy as a progressive alternative to traditional (never-ending) return-visit treatment strategies.

—Tom, 52

I started triathlons late in life at the age of 44. I soon discovered that my body was not willing to do what my determined mind wanted to do. I had sore and stiff muscles and limited range of motion in my hips and shoulders. My PT at Berman Physical Therapy explained the reasons for my problems and then gave me exercises so that these problems would not return. **I compete now in the top 15% of my age group in 30 and 70 mile races and stay healthy because of the skill and knowledge at Berman Physical Therapy.**

—Victor, 55

I am a golf professional. I also teach golf and fit golf clubs. I have been doing so in excess of 30 years. Like other golfers, I have had my "problems" with my back. I have worked with professional team Drs. No one has helped me more than Berman Physical Therapy. **Their "no frills, no pills" approach truly works.**

—Dan, 66

Berman Physical Therapy is MAGICAL!!! I'm back on the dance floor and sleeping better, too. **The medical expertise of the entire staff is unbelievable.** I will stop by someday just to give my physical therapist a hug. I can't believe how great I'm feeling.

—Lois, 63

Literally cannot say enough wonderful things about Berman Physical Therapy! I have been battling tendinitis in my right hand. I have received treatment from other physical therapists and occupational therapists—but the quality of service at Berman PT far exceeds them all. On our initial consult, my therapist asked me where I was having pain. I told him it was in my hand, and he asked, "Anywhere else?" I said, "No, nothing else really." Much to my surprise, the therapist started feeling around on my shoulders and neck. I quickly realized that much of my hand pain was a direct correlation to neck issues that I didn't even know I had. **None of my other therapists took the time to figure out the ROOT CAUSE of my pain**, they all jumped to treat what was actually hurting me at the time—which was really just a fraction of my real issues. I have likely avoided (what would have been) an inevitable hand surgery, because of their amazing knowledge and skills.

—*Jenn, 32*

Thanks to Berman Physical Therapy, **I've finally won my lifelong struggle with posture.** Hip and back pain brought me to seek help. I had been to physical therapists, chiropractors, podiatrists, and physicians, all of whom treated my symptoms, but none of whom could tell me why I had these issues to begin with, and what I could do to correct them. I learned from Berman Physical Therapy how this old body was taking the path of least resistance, but now I'm back in charge and feeling fabulous!

—*Diana, 69*

Acknowledgements

. . . .

To my wife, Jenni:

Thank you for supporting me as we travel down this wild road called life. I can't believe it's only been three years since 9/5/15! "Erry little ting is gonna be alright."

To my unborn children:

Everything I do is with you in mind. I can't wait to meet you!

To my mentor, Paul Gough:

Thank you for showing me possibilities I never thought were possible, and saving me form working harder and not smarter.

To Elizabeth Feins:

Thank you for moving this book from a dream to reality!

About The Author

. . . .

Dr. Jake Berman is the owner of Berman Physical Therapy in Naples, Florida. He graduated with highest honors from University of Florida, earning his Undergraduate Degree in Health Science before going on to finish the UF Physical Therapy Doctoral program. Dr. Berman specializes in Functional Manual Therapy, a rare form of physical therapy that uses a hands-on approach to **find problems, not just treat symptoms.**

In 2015, Dr. Berman founded Berman Physical Therapy, southwest Florida's leading outpatient PT clinic, which has helped hundreds of clients find pain relief. Berman Physical Therapy helps people age 50+ keep ACTIVE and FREE of pain meds...even if their doctors and kids are telling them to, "Just take it easy!" The clinic promotes a paradigm shift away from corporate healthcare and toward natural solutions that don't involve prescription medications or dangerous surgeries.

When he isn't hard at work treating his clients, Dr. Berman can be found golfing, fishing, or spending time with his dogs and his beautiful wife, Jenni.

Introduction:

Looking At "The Rest"

. . . .

Let me ask you a question.

That's the majority of my job, you know: asking questions.

If you were to ask my clients what I do best, they might tell you I'm good at fixing aches and pains, or that I'm a great manual physical therapist, or that I helped them avoid a dangerous surgery when every other doctor in town told them it was inescapable...but none of that is what I *do*. It's all a byproduct.

It's almost like a symptom.

This book is all about symptoms—what they are, how to interpret them, and why the most important part of my job is asking my clients about them. More than that, it's about how dangerous some symptoms can be when you zoom in close and focus on them without looking at the bigger picture.

Corporate medicine tends to operate that way—by zooming in. There's a joke about it that one of my patients, Bill, told me just last week:

A man calls up his doctor and says, "Doc, I hurt all over. It hurts when I press on my arms. It hurts when I press on my legs. It hurts when I press on my back. It even hurts when I press on my head!"

1

The doctor is baffled. He has never before encountered someone who is experiencing pain of this nature! "You'd better come into my office for an emergency appointment," the doctor says. "I'll clear my schedule for you."

When the man arrives, the doctor ushers him back to a private room.

"Now," says the doctor, "tell me again what your symptoms are."

"It's like I said, doc," says the man. "It hurts when I press on my arms. It hurts when I press on my legs. It hurts when I press on my back. It even hurts when I press on my head!"

The doctor begins examining the man. First he looks at the man's arms, and then the man's legs. He checks the man's back, and inspects the man's head. But nothing seems to be wrong!

The doctor is about to give up when he realizes there's one thing he forgot to check.

"Can you show me once more where your pain is coming from?" says the doctor.

The man points to his various body parts as he names them. "It hurts when I press on my arms, my legs, my back, and even my head. It hurts everywhere I press!"

"Sir," says the doctor, "let me see your hand."

The man holds out his hand. The doctor takes one look, and then cries, "Aha! I see what the problem is now—you've got a broken finger!"

It's a silly example, perhaps, but Bill's joke drives the point home perfectly: *the symptoms do not always tell the full story.* Imagine if the doctor in our joke had never thought to look at his

2

patient's finger. Would he have ordered expensive X-rays and MRIs? Written a prescription for painkillers? Recommended exploratory surgery on the guy's arms, legs, back, and head?

All of these options are scary, unnecessary, and more trouble than they're worth...and they're happening in real life, every single day.

It's never maliciously intended. The doctor's job is to help you get out of pain, and if you tell him that you're experiencing pain in one specific part of your body, it makes perfect sense for him to poke and prod that area. But narrowing in too closely on one part of you means that he misses the rest—and "the rest" is, in 99% of the cases I have seen in my career, the most important part.

So what's the solution?

I ask questions.

When a potential new client comes to my clinic, we generally spend the entire first visit talking. We chat about what hurts, yes, but we also discuss the more important things—things like what the client does for fun, how many grandchildren he has, which sports teams he roots for, and how many years he's been volunteering with his favorite charity. We count up all the golf games and tennis matches and fishing trips he's had to cancel because of his pain. We talk about what she would do if his problem disappeared tomorrow. We look at "the rest," because oftentimes, things that you'd never DREAM are relevant to your symptoms turn out to be the very things causing your pain.

That type of questioning doesn't happen often in any doctor's office I've ever visited.

This book is not a tirade against corporate doctors, and its goal is not to make you denounce western healthcare. It is simply going to inform—to help you understand a new way of thinking about your body, your health, and your state of mind, and perhaps to inspire you to adjust your thought process about how you determine which medical treatments you seek out for your body.

Treating symptoms is not enough. It has never been enough, and until we see a serious paradigm shift toward a healthcare system that takes "the rest" into account, it will never be enough.

So let me ask you a question: are you ready to feel better permanently?

If your answer is "YES," then this book may be the most important thing you read all year.

PART I

A Paradigm Shift

Chapter One:

What Happened To Jenni

. . . .

I didn't always feel the way I do about western medicine.

Long before I opened Berman Physical Therapy, I treated symptoms just like the rest of the doctors out there. Your knee hurts? Let's poke at it until we find the most painful point, and then massage it until it feels better. Congratulations! You're "fixed!"

The problem was, 99 patients out of 100 *weren't* fixed. The knee pain would always come back. Sure, I was providing relief in the moment, but I never addressed—or even *knew*—what was truly causing the pain. It took me years to learn that for a lot of people, knee pain can be caused by hip weakness; we can massage until the cows come home, but if we never work on strengthening those hips, the problem is always going to return.

But I didn't understand that back then. My patients wanted me to look at their knees, and I wanted to make them feel better, and that was all there was to it! It was the perfect system: I got to feel satisfied that I'd helped them, and they got to walk out pain-free... however temporarily.

Jenni changed everything.

Jenni is my beautiful wife, and her illness struck while we were dating during her first semester of physician assistant school. Jenni

9

is (and always has been) an extremely fit individual. She was a gymnast all her life, including during college, and never had any serious health issues...until one day, for no reason at all, she started having trouble keeping food in her stomach. Within minutes after eating a meal, she would have to run for the nearest bathroom. Foods she used to eat with pleasure were now causing her to become violently ill.

We attributed it to the stress of school and decided to wait it out.

Then the weight loss started.

Within six months, Jenni had dropped from a healthy 130 pounds down to an extremely unhealthy 100 pounds. One of our friends advised her to stop eating gluten, and even though there was nothing medical to back up that decision, Jenni tried it. Two weeks of gluten-free eating caused no change.

Eventually, Jenni's health had deteriorated so significantly that she was admitted to the hospital and forced to stay there for the weekend. After two full days and countless tests and blood work, we left with a diagnosis of..."dehydration." Absolutely nothing came up positive on any of her tests—she was negative for Crohn's Disease, Irritable Bowel Syndrome, celiac, and parasites. There was no reason, according to the doctors and specialists, for her inability to keep food in her system.

The Miracle Pill

We were at a loss. We tried expert after expert before we finally found a solution—a gastroenterologist named Dr. Henry who also happened to be a patient I was treating at my clinic. Dr. Henry gave Jenni every exam and test he could think of, and eventually prescribed a medication that let Jenni keep her food down for the first time in six months. To us, it seemed like a miracle—all she had to do was remember to take a pill five or ten minutes before eating a meal, and everything would go back to normal.

For the moment, it seemed we had found a cure. Jenni could eat again, although every once in awhile she forgot to take her pill before her meal, and then she'd end up right back in the bathroom. It wasn't perfect, but it was the most progress we'd had in months.

Then it shattered.

"Dr. Henry," I said to the GI during one of his visits to my clinic, "give me a Jenni update. How is she doing?"

Dr. Henry told me Jenni seemed to be improving, and that the pill was working.

"We're so relieved," I said. "How much longer do you think she'll need to be on the medication before she can go back to her regular life?"

"Hard to say," said Dr. Henry. I'll never forget what he said next: "She might be on it for the rest of her life."

The rest of her life.

The rest of her life.

"You mean the pill isn't going to fix her problem?" I said.

Dr. Henry shook his head. "Truth be told, we don't really know what the problem is. But if it's keeping the food down, then it's working, so we're just going to continue with what we know is working."

Emotions raced through my mind so quickly that I couldn't keep track of them all. Confusion. Worry. Frustration. Anger.

There was no way a normal, healthy 23-year-old woman needed to be on a medication for the rest of her life. Not without a diagnosis, anyway. Why couldn't anyone tell us the diagnosis!?

"There has to be some reason *why* this digestive issue is happening," I said.

Dr. Henry shrugged. "Sure. We can run some more tests, if you want. But they've all come up negative so far. The pill is working fine, though, isn't it?"

(At this point, whatever part of Dr. Henry I was working on—his ankle, if I recall correctly—must have been ready to snap under all the rage-fueled pressure I was using.)

"That's not the point," I said. "The point is that we're not treating the cause of the problem. We're just treating the symptoms. What is the real problem? How can somebody be perfectly normal for 22 years and then suddenly *not* be normal anymore?"

Dr. Henry shrugged again. "I just don't know."

Why We Tried Believing In Santa Claus

Jenni didn't go back to see Dr. Henry again after that. We both agreed that a doctor who "just didn't know"—a doctor who didn't even seem interested in *trying* to know—was not the type of doctor who would ever find a permanent solution for her problem.

At the time, there was an acupuncturist named Diane working out of our clinic. I had never really "bought in" to the idea of eastern medicine, but I was desperate enough for answers that I started to talk myself into it. Maybe there really was something to holistic, alternative cures—after all, eastern medicine had a 5,000-year head start on western medicine, so maybe the answer to Jenni's problem was something we westerners hadn't figured out yet. Maybe it was as simple as acupuncture. It was certainly a better option than "I don't know."

I approached Diane and asked for help understanding the eastern medicine thought process. The ideas were hard for me to grasp, especially as someone who had recently spent years of college and graduate school having the western thought process drilled into my head. Trying to believe in natural cures and alternative treatments was a little like believing in Santa Claus: it sounded *really* good, and I wanted it to be true, but I knew in my heart of hearts that it wasn't real.

(Sorry if I just ruined Santa Claus for you.)

Still, I was willing to try anything, so I nodded along with Diane's mumbo-jumbo and signed Jenni up for a few acupuncture sessions.

Jenni was even less of a believer than I was. Her PA education had ingrained western medicine philosophies into her, and it took a lot of convincing before she went to her first appointment.

No change.

Diane told us that it might take two or three sessions to start seeing a difference.

Jenni went to four. Nothing.

I wasn't ready to give up. I dove headfirst into researching eastern medicine. I found articles, watched videos, read books, studied techniques…anything I could do to find *something* resembling Jenni's case.

In the end, the answer were sitting on my bookshelf the entire time, gathering dust.

The Real Diagnosis Will SHOCK You

My aunt gave me *The Grain Brain* by Dr. David Perlmutter years ago. I'm not sure if I ever had any intention of reading it—it stayed on the top shelf of my bookcase for ages, wedged in the back where I couldn't really see it, and I didn't rediscover it until I was literally pulling out every book I owned.

I knew within the first twenty pages that I was finally, *finally* onto something. Dr. Perlmutter named countless examples of how changes in our food over the past century has led to the development of certain diseases. I'd cite the whole book here if I could—I highly recommend it to anyone who cares about nutrition, health, and wellness.

(If you don't care about any of those things, I highly recommend *The Grain Brain* anyway, because you *should* care about them, and maybe the information inside will shock you into taking care of yourself!)

I recognized elements of Jenni's symptoms on every page, and by the end of the first half of the book, I knew without a doubt that she had a gluten allergy.

"No, I don't," she said when I excitedly showed her my findings. "We already went through that."

She was technically right. Back when all of this first began, we'd tested for celiac disease. Just like everything else, it had come back negative. But after reading Dr. Perlmutter's book, I'd learned that gluten allergies have different levels of sensitivity—in order to be officially diagnosed with celiac, the patient's results have to hit a certain threshold. If Jenni was under that threshold (even if she was only *barely* under that threshold), the test would essentially ignore her sensitivity and come back negative.

It made perfect sense. She fit all the symptoms. There was a plausible explanation for how she had slipped under the radar of all her doctors. The only puzzle piece that didn't fit was the fact that when she had tried going gluten-free at the advice of a friend, she hadn't improved.

"We have to try it again," I said.

"It won't work." Jenni was just as frustrated as I was with her mystery illness, but she was far less willing to believe in my "Santa Claus" of a diagnosis. As far as she was concerned, western medicine's word was law: if all her tests had ruled out a gluten allergy, then there wasn't a gluten allergy.

"We only tried for two weeks last time," I said. "What if you can hold out for a month?"

It took so much convincing, but finally she agreed (albeit reluctantly) to cut gluten out of her diet for a month.

Just like before, there was no change during the first two weeks. Jenni still needed her pill ten minutes before each meal if she wanted to keep it down.

At the beginning of week three, she started having a little improvement—not much, but I was clinging to every shred of hope, so I celebrated. The beginning of week four was even better.

And then, on day 30, Jenni started gaining weight again.

She stopped taking her medication. As long as she avoided gluten, she didn't have any problems at mealtimes!

Fast forward to the present day. Jenni has gained almost all of her weight back, and she's in complete control of her health again. I've done my best to go gluten-free with her, although I cheat a little on the weekends, which is a luxury she doesn't have. It's very simple: if she maintains a 100% gluten-free diet, she's completely fine. If there's even the slightest cross-contamination (for example, if she cooks on a grill after someone else has used the same grill to cook something with gluten), then it's game over—straight to the bathroom.

We aren't 100% sure why Jenni's gluten allergy showed up so suddenly, but we have a pretty good guess. It all coincided with her first semester in the physician assistant program, which is an extremely stressful time—PA school squeezes the equivalent of four years of medical school into only two years, and that first semester can be a major culture shock. All of this increased stress was the "straw that broke the camel's back;" her body responded, for some reason, by refusing to tolerate gluten anymore. So the solution is...to stop eating gluten. It's that easy. It's that obvious.

Western medicine couldn't see past the tests. Western medicine meant doctor after doctor, months of poking and prodding, diagnoses of "I just don't know." Western medicine meant a lifetime of dependence on medication that was treating a symptom, not a root cause. Western medicine was *okay with never fixing Jenni's problem.*

How Everything Changed

My months of working to figure out Jenni's problem gave me a brand-new thought process when it came to treating my patients. Treating *symptoms* wasn't helping anyone; treating symptoms was like giving my wife a pill and telling her to take it before every meal for the next 80 years. In order to truly help people, I needed to give them permanent relief that wasn't dependent on a medication or a never-ending series of doctor visits. I needed to figure out what to change—be it their posture, their gait, their workout routine at the gym, or the way their hip was putting pressure on their knee—and then help them put the change into action.

Treating problems, not symptoms, is the exact thought process of functional manual therapy, and it's the philosophy I use for every client who walks into my clinic.

This book isn't about me or Jenni; it's really about you. It's part anecdote, part workbook, and part advice that will help you evaluate your own body and figure out some things your doctors have never been able to tell you. Most of all, it's going to help you —I hope—start to understand why this country desperately needs a paradigm shift away from the pill-happy, symptom-only treatments that well-intentioned (but horribly misguided) doctors keep handing out.

Chapter Two:

Neck Pain? It Could Be Your...Ankle?!

. . . .

Have you ever gone to a doctor's office and seen this question in the paperwork?

Please list all previous surgeries below

_____

_____

_____

_____

_____

_____

_____

For some reason, people like to screen their answers to this question. They leave out the surgeries that they don't think are relevant—a common question I hear in the clinic is, "I've had a lot of knee surgeries, but I'm here about my back pain, so do I really need to write all that down?"

The answer is YES.

YES, YES, YES!

The tiniest things matter when we're looking for a cure to your pain. Every surgery and injury you've ever had has affected the rest of your body in one way or another, even if the relationship isn't obvious. If I'm going to be able to treat your problems, not your symptoms, I need to be able to "zoom out"—and I can't do that effectively if I don't have all the information about "the rest" of you!

I'll give you one of my favorite examples...

The Diagnosis Scott's Doctors COMPLETELY Missed

Scott is a 68-year-old man from Naples whose neck pain was being caused by a part of the body you would never expect: his foot.

(His name isn't really Scott, by the way. In order to protect the identities of my clients, I've changed the names and identifying details of every patient whose story gets told in this book, including that GI, Dr. Henry, from the last chapter. Don't send the HIPAA police after me!)

Scott came to me in 2017 complaining about severe neck pain. "It's a herniated disc," he assured me. "I can show you the MRI."

I pried a little further—remember, the most important part of my job is asking questions! "Who told you it was a herniated disc?" I asked.

Scott looked at me like I was crazy. "It says so in my MRI."

"Who ordered the MRI?"

"My doctor. Dr. Billy Ray Bob." (The fake names strike again! Scott's doctor has a very normal name in real life.)

"And why did Dr. Billy Ray Bob order an MRI?"

I could tell Scott was getting frustrated. He knew he had a disc problem—who was I to question what his other doctor had told him?! "Because of all the pain in my neck."

"So you went in to see him," I said, "and you told him your neck hurt, and he immediately ordered an MRI?"

"Yes."

"Did he look at your hips first?"

Scott furrowed his brow. "What? Why would he look at my hips?"

I shrugged. "Scott, what do you do for fun?"

Poor Scott looked so confused! "I'm a golfer," he said finally.

I convinced him to tell me a little more about his golf habits—where he played (Kensington Golf & Country Club), how often (three times a week), how long he'd been a golfer (28 years), and whether his neck pain was affecting his golf score (yes, in a big way).

Scott told me a couple of other things during that first visit. He talked about his wife, Sheila, who liked to garden—he said he used to help her out before the neck pain started getting in the way. He and Sheila were very adventurous. They took an African safari for their honeymoon, and on their 25th wedding anniversary they went skiing in the Alps. Scott wanted to surprise her with a trip to Thailand for her 65th birthday, but he was worried about trying to travel in all this pain.

"I think it needs surgery," he said. "That's what Dr. Billy Ray Bob said. I just wanted a second opinion before I scheduled anything."

"Stand up," I said. "I want to take a look at your hips."

Scott looked a little exasperated, but he did what I asked. "I've never had a problem with my hips," he said. "It's my neck."

"How did you hurt your neck?" I asked.

"It's a herniated disc."

"No, I mean, what did you do? Did you fall? Did you twist it a certain way?"

"Oh." Scott paused. "I don't think so. It just sort of happened."

"When?"

"I'm not sure. It's been there for years."

"Hm." I put Scott in a variety of positions, all designed to test out his hip strength. "Walk to the other side of the treatment room for me."

He did. There was a very significant sway to the way he walked; one hip was always cocked a little higher than the other, as if he was favoring his right side. The crookedness continued all the way up his body. One shoulder was dropped, and his head was tilted very slightly to one side—the perfect recipe for poor posture, and in turn, neck pain!

"Have you ever had any trauma in your hip area?" I asked.

He shook his head.

"What about your knees? Or your feet?"

He thought for a moment. "I broke my left ankle a long time ago," he said. "Probably 40 years ago. It was during the physical test to join the police academy—I really wanted to be a police officer when I was in college. I tripped and fell, and my ankle snapped."

It was all starting to come together. "Did you need surgery?"

"Yes. There are a couple of screws holding it together."

Aha! He hadn't written that surgery down on his paperwork!

"Did you go to physical therapy to rehab your ankle?" I asked him.

Scott thought about it for a second. "I think so. They gave me some exercises to do. I didn't really do them. Once I could walk, I didn't think there was a point."

I nodded. "Let me see you walk again."

Stand up right now yourself and try taking a few steps in slow motion. Feel how your weight shifts from foot to foot. Notice the way you push off with the toes, flexing the back foot. It should all happen very fluidly, without stiffness.

Scott's walk was not fluid. His left ankle and foot looked significantly stiffer than his right—a telltale sign of someone who didn't re-learn how to walk the right way! His toes didn't push off, creating the slightest limp, and the rest of his body was compensating by tilting off-center, which was making his posture crooked.

Poor posture is probably the number one cause of pain I see in my clinic—neck pain included—and now that I could see Scott had been practicing bad posture ever since his ankle injury 40 years ago, I knew we had found the reason for his symptoms.

"Let's work on the ankle," I said.

How Your MRI Could Be Fooling You

Scott was resistant, as I knew he would be. "It's not my ankle that's the problem! It's the herniated disc in my neck. Can you just tell me if I'm going to need surgery or not?"

I explained my entire thought process to Scott: how yes, there *was* a herniated disc, but that zooming in too closely on the MRI results meant that we would miss key details. This is a conversation I have a lot with clients who have grown up surrounded by the western medical process.

And I don't blame them. Having a medical scan is a very complex, scary process to go through, and the average person doesn't understand how it works or what the results mean. That's why you can't "read" your own MRI—you have to go to your doctor and have him or her interpret it for you. You might know some buzzwords, the way Scott knew that a "herniated disc" was a bad thing, but when I ask people to explain to me what a herniated disc *is,* a lot of times they're at a loss. They have no choice but to rely on what their doctors tell them, because they don't have a medical education that will allow them to draw their own conclusions.

There are, of course, exceptions. I've treated all kinds of doctors, nurses, and other medical professionals who know exactly what they're talking about—and I've also seen a lot of people without formal medical training who have done their research. But for the most part, the clients I work with are completely overwhelmed by the medical jargon their doctors throw around. They trust what the MRI says because they don't know any better —just like Jenni and I used to trust the negative celiac test and the miracle pill before we found Dr. Perlmutter's book.

"But how can my MRI be wrong?" Scott asked. "It's right there. Dr. Billy Ray Bob wrote that I have herniation."

He was right. There was a herniation, and the MRI wasn't

edited or misinterpreted. But what a lot of people don't know is that herniated discs don't always cause pain.

I'll say it again, because it's very important.

Herniated discs do not always cause pain.

One more time, for the people in the back:

HERNIATED DISCS DO NOT ALWAYS CAUSE PAIN!

There was a study done recently on a group of more than 1,000 asymptomatic people over age 60. "Asymptomatic" means that the people who volunteered for this study had no symptoms—no back pain, no neck pain, no history of disc problems, no health issues of any kind. The participants were all given MRIs, and then a team of experts interpreted the imaging. The results were astounding: 60% of the MRIs showed disc problems! Herniations, bulges, slipped discs…these people's spines were a mess!

Yet for some reason, everyone was asymptomatic. The disc issues were real, but they weren't causing any pain.

How does this apply to someone like Scott?

Well, Scott told me that he had never had an MRI done prior to the one on his neck.

That means that the disc could have been herniated for his entire adult life without causing a problem—we have no way of knowing when it first ruptured, because we have no older MRIs to study and compare. If Scott was one of those people whose disc problem causes no pain (and there's a 60% chance that he was, based on that study!), then focusing on his disc would be a waste of time.

It would be like putting a band-aid on your *left* knee after scraping up your *right* knee. Sure, you bandaged up your knee…

but you didn't do anything effective! Fixing something that doesn't hurt is *never* going to cure your pain.

I explained all of this to Scott. He still wasn't ready to buy in. "What if I'm not the 60%?" he asked. "What if it really *is* my herniated disc causing the pain?"

That's a fair question. "Working on a disc is a lot more serious than working on posture," I said. "Let's start with the ankle. The ankle will fix your posture, and if your pain goes away after that, then we can congratulate ourselves on avoiding surgery. If your pain doesn't go away, the herniated disc will still be there for us to work on. How does that sound?"

Scott said it sounded okay.

Six weeks later, he was discharged from my clinic with perfect posture and no more pain.

We never *once* worked on his neck.

He sent me a postcard from Thailand.

10 Important Things Your MRI Won't Show You

So here we are again, back at the issue of doctors who zoom in too far. Dr. Billy Ray Bob didn't truly examine Scott—as soon as he heard that "neck pain" was the symptom, he focused in on the neck! He ordered the MRI, searched for anything that *might* be causing pain, and then presented his findings as if there was a 100% chance that the disc was the problem.

But as you now know, more than half the time, pain like Scott's is caused by factors that medical scans can't see. Factors like:

1. Poor posture
2. Nerve entrapment
3. Strained ligaments
4. Joint capsule restrictions
5. Core instability
6. Muscle imbalance
7. SI joint dysfunctions
8. Hip instability
9. Pelvic obliquities
10. Hip capsule restrictions

Here, I'll even throw in four more "bonus" factors that MRIs can't see:

11. Fascial restrictions
12. Diaphragm issues
13. Pelvis floor issues
14. Using improper workout techniques

...and that's just conditions I've treated in the past week!

Scott is actually one of the lucky ones. There's another client I saw in 2017, Deb, who presented a very similar case: back pain was interrupting her active lifestyle, making it impossible to travel or play the sport she loved (in her case, it was pickleball). The difference was that Deb's MRI did *not* show any disc herniation, and so her doctor, Dr. Billy Ray Joe, was at a loss for how to treat her.

"He gave me a prescription for pain meds," Deb said when I

talked to her at her first appointment. "It was a month's supply of pills. I felt really good when I was taking them, but as soon as they wore off, the pain came back."

Deb went back to Dr. Billy Ray Joe month after month to get refills for her prescription. She told me she hated being on pills, but her life was "agony" without them. Dr. Billy Ray Joe coached Deb through chiropractic treatments, massage therapy, steroid injections, and even an epidural, but nothing helped for very long.

"The chiropractor told me I was out of alignment, but when he adjusted me, it would just make my back feel worse, so I stopped going there." Deb sighed. "Eventually, we were out of options. I had some exploratory surgery, but they didn't find anything."

Exploratory surgery!

"I'm just at a loss. Dr. Billy Ray Joe says the next step is neurolysis. Isn't that where they go in and burn off your nerves so you stop feeling pain?"

Yes, that's exactly what neurolysis is: the cauterization of nerves and pain receptors. It's the ultimate "I don't know" diagnosis—the doctors can't fix your problem because they can't figure out your problem, so they just burn off your pain receptors, as if ignoring the pain will magically make the issue go away.

It's like taking the world's largest pain pill.

People who go through with neurolysis treatments end up doing *untold* damage to their bodies. They can't feel pain anymore in their problem area, so they assume they're "fixed," and they go back to living the active lives they couldn't have before when the pain was too intense. Meanwhile, their problem areas—which are *still problem areas*, even if they can't feel it anymore—get worse and worse, and they have no idea.

And by the way, **neurolysis isn't permanent!** Over time, the body will repair and regenerate the cauterized nerves, so the pain will slowly come back...and this time, it's even worse than before, because of all the activity the person has been pushing themselves to do while they were pain-free.

So what did I say to Deb?

You can probably guess: "Let me take a look at your hips."

Deb's problem was, like the chiropractor had noticed, an issue of alignment. But adjustments weren't the way to go; Deb needed to strengthen her hip muscles so she could support herself on her own. She had been playing pickleball for years with weak hips, and to compensate for all the physical activity, she was walking slightly crooked without even realizing it. Just like Scott, her posture was poor—and it was as simple as that.

It took about two months, but when Deb was discharged from my clinic, she walked out the door with completely stable hips and no pain in her back.

I followed up with her recently when I asked if I could use her story for this book, and she told me she hasn't needed a pain pill in more than a year.

How To Avoid Doctors, Pain Meds, Surgeries, Neurolysis, And All That Other Stuff...Starting TODAY

What does this mean for you?

It means that if you ever have an "impossible" problem that baffles doctors and mystifies specialists, you might need to step back from the western medicine thought process for a moment.

Find a doctor who is willing to look your whole body and your whole history—I'll save you a lot of time and tell you that the best kind of doctor for this is a physical therapist. Don't let anyone zoom in on your problem area, or get caught up in your symptoms. Refuse to let the MRI results be the be-all and end-all of your diagnosis.

The second half of this book is a guide to common causes of aches and pains that a lot of doctors miss. You can use those chapters to help you; skip ahead to the chapter about your type of pain, and I'll give you the following:

1. A list of reasons you might hurt (that WON'T show up in an MRI)

2. Solutions that you can put into action immediately, in the comfort of your own home, that will stop your pain in its tracks

3. Exercises, at-home tests, self-evaluations, and more that will help you begin to diagnose yourself

4. Resources beyond this book that will help your road to recovery, including links to access my exclusive YouTube videos, reports, monthly newsletters, and health/fitness blog posts

5. Explicit instructions on how to qualify for a complimentary Discovery Visit at Berman Physical Therapy, so you can hear what our specialists have to say about your problem— absolutely free of charge

Chapter Three:

The Shocking Reason Medicare Is Harming Your Health

* *

I want to share a secret with you that a truly astounding number of people don't know:

Your insurance is ruining your health.

This is the case for most insurance companies, but it's *especially* true for Medicare.

90% of my clients have Medicare, and they're all very surprised the first time they hear my stance on it. One client, Leslie, was especially shocked. "Medicare covers *everything*," she told me. "How can you tell me it's bad?"

To answer that, we have to take a look at what physical therapy was like back in the 1980s and early 1990s. That was the heyday of physical therapy. If I'd been practicing back then, I would have been able to see one patient per hour, bill the patient's insurance company my rate, and be fully reimbursed for my services.

Then the HMOs came out—that's "Health Maintenance Organization," and it's the type of insurance plan that only pays for patients to see doctors who are "in network"—and Medicare changed its policy to reimburse only a *percentage* of what was billed for physical therapy services. All the other insurance companies followed suit and did the same.

That was the beginning of the end for quality service in the medical field. Because of the decrease in reimbursement rates, physical therapists have to drastically increase the volume of patients they see every day—otherwise they won't be able to get enough reimbursement money from the insurance companies to keep keep their doors open.

Now, when you have to squeeze in too many patients per day, it becomes extremely difficult to provide quality hands-on manual therapy. Working one-on-one with a patient for one hour is ideal; if I had to cut that hour in half, I would lose *extremely* valuable time. I wouldn't be able to ask questions anymore, which means I would never get to figure out the root cause of most symptoms, and I would rarely be able to cure anybody. I would be right back where I started: treating symptoms. And, as I've witnessed time and time again, treating symptoms never permanently fixes anyone.

It gets worse. Half an hour is enough time to do *some* hands-on manual therapy, and with enough appointments, I'd be able to figure out the problem and make progress. But most offices can't even afford to let their physical therapists spend half an hour with each patient! With Medicare reimbursing for physical therapy at such low rates, clinics—especially clinics in southwest Florida, where the majority of patients are using Medicare—have no choice but to book their PTs with *three or four* patients per hour. That means that if you're using your Medicare to pay for physical therapy appointments, you could spend as little as fifteen minutes working directly with your physical therapist!

Now, scheduling all those appointments (up to 32 clients per therapist per day!) is a clerical nightmare. If the clinic employs multiple physical therapists, you're probably not going to get to choose one that you like and stick with that person—you'll be bounced around from PT to PT, and the only thing they'll know about your problem is whatever the last PT scribbled down in your file as he rushed from patient to patient.

After you spend your fifteen minutes with the physical therapist who barely knows what's wrong with you, you'll probably be handed off to a tech or an assistant. It's the same situation: the assistant is exhausted from working with three or four patients per hour, and has very little idea who you are and why you're in physical therapy to begin with. You'll probably be handed a list of exercises to work on while the assistant supervises (or runs to check on another patient). These might be exercises you have no idea how to do, or they might be exercises you only *think* you know how to do—and if you try to do them with incorrect form, you run the risk of hurting yourself even more.

Here's where things get even more shocking—my client, Leslie, couldn't believe her ears when I told her this next part!

Medicare pays different rates for different treatment codes. That means that Medicare considers certain services more expensive than others, and so it sends the clinic more money if the physical therapist completes those services.

So what do you think happens?

The physical therapists are strongly encouraged to complete the services that will generate more revenue—*even if those services are not right for the patients!*

What In-Network "Cookie Cutter" Physical Therapy Is Actually Like

One of my clients, Anne, came to see me after wasting months on this type of "cookie cutter" physical therapy—we call it "cookie cutter" because the treatment plan you get is always the same, no matter what unique nuances are involved in your specific case. Anne had a shoulder impingement syndrome, and she was trying to avoid surgery. She chose her first physical therapy office based on the recommendation of her orthopedic surgeon, who owned the PT clinic.

Anne described her treatment to me. "There was a machine that looked like a bike, but you pedaled it with your hands. I had to use that for fifteen minutes. Then they had me reach up over my head and pull on a pulley system for five minutes. I did all that in a room by myself. It was *so* boring. I used to stare out the window and count the cars driving past the office. After that, the PT came in and did ten minutes of massage and ten minutes of electric stim. Then they had me do twenty minutes of ice."

This is a classic "cookie cutter" appointment. Notice how much time Anne got to spend receiving hands-on treatment (ten minutes of massage) compared to how much time she had to spend on her own (50 minutes doing unsupervised exercises on machines or using modalities). At the time of this book's publication, Medicare pays more for therapeutic exercise than for manual therapy, so physical therapists often try to have their clients do as much exercise as possible, and they limit the manual, hands-on treatment.

An appointment like Anne's has nothing to do with a client's well-being and *everything* to do with a clinic desperately trying to make money from insurance reimbursement! Generic exercises and modalities are much less effective than hands-on therapy by a professional—*especially* when those generic exercises are unsupervised, and there's a chance the patient is doing them wrong!

"How long did it take you to get better?" I asked Anne.

Anne thought about it for a moment. "I probably went four or five times before my orthopedic surgeon said it wasn't effective."

"Did you try a different physical therapist?" I asked.

"No," Anne said. "I had the surgery. Afterwards, I went back for my post-op physical therapy at the same place."

I asked Anne why she went back to the same clinic after her surgery when it hadn't helped before.

"They already had my insurance on file." Anne shrugged. "It seemed easier to stay with what I knew, I guess."

"So how long did you go to them this time?" I asked.

"I went three times a week for three or four weeks. Then my shoulder froze and I had to stop physical therapy altogether."

"What kind of treatment did they give you this time?"

"It didn't change. I did the hand-peddling on the bike, the pulley, ten minutes of massage, and then some stim and ice."

"Just to clarify," I said, "your treatment after surgery was exactly the same as your treatment before surgery?"

Anne nodded. "Honestly, I think they do the same thing for everyone with shoulder problems."

Anne was right. Having "cookie cutter" physical therapy means that nothing is customized; with up to 32 patients per day, the PTs don't have *time* to customize! There's no time to stop and ask questions, or to figure out what's *really* wrong, or to do anything but treat the symptoms.

I've worked in offices that operated that way. I knew exactly what Anne was talking about.

About three years later, Anne's other shoulder started showing the same impingement symptoms. Fearing another surgery (and another frozen shoulder!), she chose not to go back to her orthopedic surgeon or her original physical therapy office. She started asking around town for a physical therapist who could actually address her problem—and she now knew what kind of questions to ask in order to find someone effective. She knew she wanted to see a physical therapist for more than ten minutes, and she knew she needed more hands-on treatment and less of the boring, mindless exercises.

Her questions led her to Berman Physical Therapy, where she spent a total of three visits working one-on-one with a shoulder specialist.

At each appointment, he spent a full hour delivering hands-on treatment to restore her range of motion and eliminate the impingement. He also gave her a list of three "homework" exercises that would strengthen the shoulder—and he made sure she knew exactly how to do each exercise before he prescribed them.

"He even took videos on my phone so I would remember everything," Anne said. "It was such a different experience."

How long did it take to fix Anne's shoulder this time?

"Three visits." Anne stretched her arm over her head to demonstrate her full range of motion. "No more surgery for me."

How To Afford Out-Of-Network Costs

I explained all of this to Leslie, giving her a complete breakdown of the ways Medicare is harmful to the health of patients, including:

- How its low reimbursement rates force physical therapists to carry huge case loads they can't maintain...

- How this huge case loads result in "cookie cutter" physical therapy, because there's no time to ask the right questions about symptoms, and so the physical therapists are forced to treat every injury the same way...

- How Medicare's inconsistent rates incentivize the prescription of "exercise" instead of quality, hands-on physical therapy...

- How these inconsistent rates *also* result in physical therapists giving out treatments that won't even help their patients, just because the clinic owner needs to increase revenue to keep the lights on!

When I was finished, Leslie *still* wasn't convinced! "Medicare covers everything," she said to me. "Money is a big factor for me. I just can't afford to pay out-of-network costs."

That's completely understandable. I have piles of debt from grad school that I'm trying to pay off, so I know how difficult it can be to justify big purchases—especially big purchases that I could get somewhere else for free!

Here's what I told Leslie to do: take some time to think about what she valued the most. Was it money? Was it her health? Was it tennis, which she had played all her life up until a shoulder injury made her stop? (That was why she was in my office—just like Anne, she wanted to use physical therapy to avoid a shoulder surgery.)

If money was truly the most important thing on that list, I told her, then I wanted her to put the money first and find a solution that involved using Medicare. But if health or tennis was first on her list, then she should allow herself to spend a little money on out-of-network services.

"It's completely up to you," I said. "I won't question your priorities. If you need to put money ahead of health and tennis, then that's what you need to do. I just want to make sure you have all the information, and that you know in your heart that you're making the right decision."

Leslie promised to call me if she chose anything other than money.

The phone rang the next morning, and she booked her first appointment.

Five Questions The Other Guys DON'T Want You Asking

After hearing about Anne's experience, I decided to create a list of questions that will help you determine whether a clinic offers "cookie cutter" physical therapy or quality, hands-on manual therapy that is customized to your needs and will actually treat your problems, not your symptoms.

Take a break from this book to call a few places—you can Google "best physical therapy in Naples" (or wherever you live!) for ideas—and fill out the form on the next page accordingly:

Five Questions The Other Guys Don't Want You Asking

1. How much one-on-one time will I spend with my physical therapist (NOT a tech or an assistant) during my initial evaluation and follow-up appointments?

LOCATION	INITIAL EVALUATION	FOLLOW-UPS
1. Berman PT	60 minutes	60 minutes
2.		
3.		

2. What is the maximum number of people each physical therapist sees per hour?

LOCATION	MAXIMUM # OF PATIENTS
1. Berman PT	We see one patient per hour
2.	
3.	

3. What are the qualifications of the technicians/assistants that I will be working with?

LOCATION	QUALIFICATIONS
1. Berman PT	We don't use technicians or assistants
2.	
3.	

4. Will I have the same therapist every visit?

LOCATION	SAME THERAPIST?
1. Berman PT	Yes, unless you request otherwise
2.	
3.	

5. Do your therapists perform manual therapy or hands-on treatment at every visit?

LOCATION	HANDS-ON AT EVERY APPOINTMENT?
1. Berman PT	Yes; we never use modalities
2.	
3.	

If you're like Leslie and you put money high up on your list of things you value, here's a bonus question you can ask:

6. Do you offer any kind of Satisfaction Guarantee?

LOCATION	GUARANTEE
1. Berman PT	Yes; if you aren't happy with your treatment, we refund 100%
2.	
3.	

Chapter Four:

Ten Things You Didn't Know Your Physical Therapist Could Help You With

. . . .

Here's a crazy "small world" story that goes around our office every once in awhile.

One of our office admins, Elizabeth, has extremely painful bunions: bony bumps that formed on the joints at the base of her big toes. She used to be a gymnast, but the pain in her feet—especially the right one—forced her to give up her sport when she was only nine years old.

By age 13, she and her mom were driving all over southwest Florida for surgical consultations.

At age 15, she had a bunionectomy on her right foot...and then went for her post-op physical therapy *right here in our office!*

Now, this was several years ago, before Berman Physical Therapy existed. Back then, our office belonged to a different, "cookie cutter" physical therapy clinic. And the treatment Elizabeth had there was so ineffective that she never got her foot back to its full range of motion, and she still experiences numbness and nerve pain along her surgery scar.

Who would have thought that she'd end up working in the very same building nearly a decade later!?

Here's the thing: Elizabeth thought her only option was surgery.

If you Google "bunion cure," that's really the only solution that the Internet suggests. There are braces and orthotics that can buy you time (we'll chat in a later chapter about why all that stuff actually makes foot pain WORSE), but ultimately, the only long-term options you'll find online are invasive procedures.

What if I told you physical therapy could cure bunions just as effectively as surgery?

When I told Elizabeth, she was skeptical. But she let one of our PTs work on her left foot—which still had a bunion, because she only had surgery on the right foot—and was shocked to find that her restricted range of motion was almost completely restored after just one quick session!

Decreasing her pain was just a matter of learning how to engage different foot muscles when she was walking or standing, and a week later she was reporting significant improvements.

That physical therapy we helped Elizabeth go through was a lot less expensive, dangerous, and time-consuming than surgery, but more than that, it got to the root of her problem. The problem was never her bunions, or even her pain—the problem was that she was using the wrong muscles when she walked.

Everything else was just a symptom.

The best bunionectomy in the world won't teach you how to utilize different muscles, and so it was never the right fix for Elizabeth.

The Ten (Extremely Treatable) Conditions You Would NEVER Think To Call A Physical Therapist About

You won't see very many PT clinics advertising that they fix bunions.

In fact, there are a lot of conditions we treat that you wouldn't normally associate with physical therapy.

Physical therapy isn't the kind of thing most people send themselves to. Most people—not all of them, but *most* of them— think physical therapy is just for recovering from injuries or surgeries. If you have chronic pain that doesn't seem to be related to anything you did recently, chances are, you're going to head straight to your general practitioner, or start asking around for a back/knee/neck/hip/anything else specialist in your area.

It's very rare that I run into a client who says, "Physical therapy was my first thought as soon as I realized I was in pain!" So if that's you, congratulations on being one of the few!

If you're like most people, however, you probably didn't realize physical therapists can help with aches and pains unrelated to traumas.

So I came up with a list of ten things you probably didn't know a physical therapist can help you with.

In no particular order, here they are:

1. Migraines/headaches
2. Vertigo
3. TMJ
4. Chronic pain that has been there for years

5. Scoliosis
6. The inability to play with your grandkids
7. Balance
8. Your golf game
9. Sleeping better
10. Osteoarthritis

Did any of those surprise you? Usually people giggle when we say we can help their golf game...but the majority of our clients are golfers (or some other type of athlete—runners, tennis players, even pickleballers!) who can't play as effectively as they want to because some kind of physical restriction is holding them back!

Many of these ten conditions will be addressed in Part II of this book, which is titled "Head To Toe" and serves as a guide to common causes of aches and pains. In that section, I'll dive a little more deeply into the scientific side of why you might be hurting, and what you can do to fix it.

For now, though, as we explore this list of ten conditions you didn't know PT could help, we'll keep everything nice and simple, so that absolutely anyone can understand it.

Read on for #1!

1. Migraines/Headaches

· ·

Everyone gets a headache once in awhile, but if you're experiencing chronic headaches that show up frequently and stay for days, there could be a physical problem causing them. The go-to solution that most doctors provide is either:

A) Prescription painkillers

or

B) Brain scans

While it's never a bad idea to check on the brain, especially after a traumatic injury, the vast majority of these scans come up negative. So once you know there's nothing wrong with your brain, it's time to explore other options.

Headaches can be related to diet—if you aren't getting enough nutrients, or if you're often dehydrated, that could be causing the problem.

But usually, by the time people with chronic headaches and migraines think to call us, they've already been through all that. They feel desperate and hopeless—they tell us that the specialists can't figure out what's wrong with them, and they see physical therapy as a last resort before they resign themselves to a life of pain (and pain medication!).

You might be surprised to learn that the solutions we discover for these people are often EXTREMELY simple. It's not that headaches are too complicated for doctors to figure out—it's that the doctors are so busy rushing between patients that they can't take the time to look at the whole body! It's easier and faster to order a CT scan, a PET scan, an MRI, a series of blood tests, or a prescription medication...at least, it's easier and faster *for the doctor.* For the patient, it's a much more difficult process that involves time out of your day, money out of your wallet, and the extra stress of not knowing whether any of these things will work.

Here's where physical therapy comes in.

If there's any kind of pattern to your headaches—for example, if you notice that you always get headaches when you turn your head to one side, or if a migraine tends to show up when you sit in the same position for a long time—then there's a good chance they're being caused by something muscular! Things like tense neck muscles and poor posture can contribute heavily to headaches. If you're the type of person who is easily stressed, your muscles will automatically become tenser, making your headaches last longer and occur more frequently.

Something as vague as "tension" will never show up in a brain scan or blood test, but a manual physical therapist will know within minutes whether your headaches are muscle-based!

So what's the next step? We'll loosen up the muscles that are causing the tension by mobilize your joints and focusing on your posture. Generally, this is enough to dramatically decrease the severity of migraines, and it can cure chronic headaches altogether!

How We Cured Chip's Headaches With One VERY Easy Trick

One of my recent clients, Chip, came to Berman Physical

Therapy complaining of severe headaches whenever he drove. Chip worked for a limousine service and often drove for 10–12 hours per day. His headaches were interfering with his ability to work—every shift was "like torture," and he was seriously considering leaving his job.

The solution was almost hilariously simple: the drivers seat in Chip's limo was too far back! He had to lean forward to reach the steering wheel, resulting in terrible posture and extremely stiff joints. All of this, combined with the stress of coming to work for his daily "torture," was causing Chip to tense up his shoulders and neck, which restricted the blood flow to his brain and caused headaches.

All it took to fix Chip's posture was adjusting his seat to bring it closer to the steering wheel. His headaches disappeared almost immediately; we worked with him on his posture for a few sessions, and then we sent him on his merry way.

No brain scan in the world will show you that your car seat is positioned wrong! Chip had been to several doctors—and given up several work shifts in order to make it to those appointments—but not one of them had asked what he did for a living, or what kinds of activities brought on his headaches. It took a physical therapist who *cared enough to ask the right questions* to help Chip get out of pain.

If you're at the end of your rope with "headache specialists," consider physical therapy for headache needs.

(Keep reading for #2…)

2. Vertigo

. . . .

Remember when you used to do cartwheels or spin around as fast as you could when you were a kid? Back when getting dizzy and falling over was something you did for FUN?

Ah, the good old days!

If you suffer from vertigo, then you've experienced that "Alice in Wonderland" effect, where the room feels like it's rotating, rocking, or spinning around you, even when you're standing perfectly still. It usually induces lightheadedness, nausea, or vomiting—and each episode can last for hours or even days!

You may already know that vertigo has something to do with the inner ear. The ear is a very complicated system, but let's focus on the basics: your ear is made up of three semi-circular "canals."

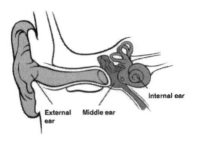

As fluid circulates through the canals, the brain is able to detect your body movement and help you feel grounded and centered. As you age, however, and you stop a lot of the activities you used to do (like cartwheels and spinning!), the fluid starts having trouble circulating. And when the fluid doesn't circulate, the brain doesn't know how to interpret your body movement, which results in vertigo and general dizziness!

Doctors generally recommend medication and steroid shots to treat vertigo-related dizziness, but as we've discussed again and again, writing a prescription to alleviate a symptom is *never* going to cure the root cause!

A good physical therapist can completely resolve vertigo in just a few sessions. Using specific maneuvers that involve tilting the head in certain patterns, we can clear out the inner ear canals and get that fluid flowing freely again! It's quick and natural—and because it addresses the root cause of your dizziness, it won't "wear off" like a pain pill or injection, which is only serving to mask the vertigo.

(The next condition you didn't know PT could help is jaw-dropping! Keep reading for #3!)

3. TMJ Dysfunctions

• •

"TMJ" is the abbreviation for "temporomandibular joint," which is the technical term for "that hinge where your jaw mets your cheekbone." If the hinge ever comes out of alignment, it can lock up (keeping your mouth clamped closed *or* stuck wide open) and cause extreme discomfort.

People usually call up their dental offices when they discover a TMJ dysfunction, but the best a dentist can do is fit you with a mouth guard to wear at night. This type of treatment rarely has an "end date;" the longer you wear them, the more you'll come to depend on them.

If and when the mouth guard fails to solve the problem, a lot of TMJ-sufferers turn to medications. Muscle relaxers can take away the pain, but they are highly addictive, and generally do more harm than good—and like all medications, they only "mask" the pain, addressing a symptom instead of a problem!

Some people choose surgery. One of our clients told us she tried botox injections to relax the joint and slide it back into place, but the painful (and expensive) treatment was completely ineffective.

I rarely see physical therapy clinics (besides our own office!) advertising that they can fix a TMJ dysfunction, but it's really no different from treating any other joint problem! A great TMJ client success story is Brian, a 72-year-old man who came to us after a major jaw surgery. The surgery didn't directly involve the TMJ, but after weeks of having his jaw wired shut while it healed, he had lost all mobility in the hinge area. Now that he was unwired, the joint kept slipping out of alignment.

Using the same techniques we use on other tight muscles, we relaxed Brian's TMJ muscles to allow proper motion. We also taught him strengthening exercises so that he could hold his jaw in the proper position. Finally, we addressed his posture—if you tend to slouch or hunch your shoulders, you might notice that your chin juts out, creating an underbite and straining your jaw muscles. Fixing that posture helps align the jaw, which in turn decreases the TMJ dysfunction.

If your jaw ever gets stuck in a painful position, try physical therapy before you head to the dentist. Chances are, you'll have more luck in our office!

(Think you're just in pain because you're "old?" #4 will prove that that's NOT true!)

4. Chronic pain that's been there for years (or even decades)

• •

There's a myth going around Naples that being in pain is just part of getting old.

But think about it—there are people out there in their 60s, 70s, 80s, and even 90s who are living extremely active lives without pain! Just Google "90-year-old marathon runners." You'll be shocked by how many articles come up!

If pain really were an inevitable part of aging, would people *older than you* be living pain-free? No! But they are.

I can tell you exactly how that "old age = pain" myth got started.

Let's say that as a child, you used to eat a triple-scoop ice cream cone every single day. You continued to eat your triple-scoop every single day, without fail, all the way through your teens, your 20s, your 30s...all the way up to your 80s! By this point, you've had an extremely unhealthy diet for DECADES—so it shouldn't come as a surprise that you're experiencing health complications, like obesity or diabetes.

How ridiculous would it sound if your doctor said, "Being diabetic is just a part of growing older?" Of course that's not true! There are tons of people in their 80s without diabetes! Your health problems are happening because you practiced a bad habit—eating triple-scoops of ice cream almost 30,000 days in a row—and the side effects have been slowly catching up for 80 years.

The same concept applies to "chronic" pain. If you have an ache that built up gradually for no apparent reason, it's probably the side effects of practicing a bad habit for years. Maybe you worked at a job that required you to hunch over a desk, and now your neck, shoulders, and back are paying the price for using poor posture over the years. Maybe you always balanced your children on the same side of your body when you picked them up as babies, and the hip on that side is finally starting to feel the effects.

Whatever the specific area of your pain, I guarantee there's a cause BESIDES your age.

What Will Happen If You Don't Find That Cause

Now, let's take this a step further and look into the future for a moment.

If your "old age" pain becomes bad enough that it limits the things you love to do—golf, tennis, walking on the beach, playing with your grandchildren, or whatever else your favorite hobbies may be—you have two choices. You can "deal with it" and lose the activities you love, or you can visit a medical professional.

If you choose a physical therapist who knows how to treat problems, not symptoms, you're going to have a lot of success! But unfortunately, a lot of people *just don't realize* that PT can help with chronic pain. Those people choose their regular doctors—they don't know any better.

You know the rest: the doctors are stretched thin because they need to see as many patients as possible, so they can bill as many insurance companies as possible, so they can make money. They only get to spend a few minutes with you—not enough time to figure out the root problem of your pain—so they write you a prescription for pain medications, order a few X-rays or MRIs, and send you off to a surgeon.

What would you do if you went through a major spinal surgery and later found out that you could have cured your back pain naturally just by slightly adjusting your posture?

How would you feel if you had a hip replacement and discovered afterwards that it could have been avoided if you'd just started balancing your grandkids on the other side when you picked them up?

This is the type of story we hear ALL THE TIME!

Now, for some people, chronic pain can be the result of a traumatic injury or surgery. Anything that leaves behind scar tissue is going to cause complications later on. I can't tell you how many clients I've seen who tell me they broke their arm or leg 20 years ago and it still causes them pain because it "never healed properly." 99% of the time, it healed just fine—it's the *scar tissue* that's causing the pain!

Why Scar Tissue Could Secretly Be The Cause Of Your Pain

When you acquire scar tissue, everything under the surface starts to thicken up and become immobile. There's a lot going on in the space between your skin and your muscle, and each layer of tissue needs to "slide and glide" on top of each other in order to move properly; scar tissue makes things sticky, and so the nerves trying to navigate through the tissue become stuck. If you notice any tingling or loss of sensation along a scar, that's probably a trapped nerve!

Want to hear the craziest part?

There are people—some of them are clients of mine—who visit their doctors to have their scar tissue checked out...*and they end up having surgery to remove the scar tissue!*

Of course, the surgery results in even *more* scar tissue, which means more pain, more frustration, and more hopelessness. A good physical therapist, like the ones in our office, will know hands-on, non-surgical techniques that will break down the scar tissue and free up all those other layers of tissue.

If everything else you've tried has been ineffective for your chronic pain, consider physical therapy. It could be the miracle cure you've been searching for!

(Is your back pain "untreatable" without surgery? #5 will show you a secret cure!)

5. Scoliosis

· ·

Scoliosis (that's pronounced skoh-lee-OH-sis!) is a condition that makes your spine curve, like the letter S. Unsurprisingly, this contributes heavily to back pain!

There are some people, though it's extremely rare, who are born with scoliosis, but for most people scoliosis is something you acquire over time. If one hip is weaker than the other, you're likely to stand with all your weight on one side, which will force your spine to bend out of alignment in order to keep you balanced. Over time, as you "train" the spine to overcompensate, the bend becomes permanent.

But, like the other chronic pains that build up over time, scoliosis is treatable without resorting to drastic measures like surgery—if you find the right physical therapist, that is!

One of my recent clients, Janice, has the PERFECT scoliosis success story! Janice is a 53-year-old female who was extremely active in her youth. She ran track and cross country in middle school, she joined the swim team in high school, and she was on her college's varsity rowing team. She has always loved working out and staying fit.

Being as intensely athletic as Janice is comes with a few injuries and surgeries along the way, but she told me she has a high tolerance for pain, and that she has learned to ignore some of her body's warning signs because she doesn't want to seem like a "wimp."

After college, Janice stopped playing most of her sports, but she continued to stay active with fitness classes. She currently goes to barre classes at least four mornings per week before she heads off to her job as a teacher.

Now, Janice is the mother of four children, two of whom are twins. Her pregnancies caused a lot of stress on her body, especially her lower back.

She also experiences a lot of pain in her left hip. That's common in mothers, because they tend to hold their babies on the same side of their bodies every time, which puts a lot of pressure on one hip.

Janice's position of comfort is turned to the right and bent to the left. When she bends down, her right side sticks up further than her left—a telltale sign of scoliosis!

It was the scoliosis that finally caused Janice to seek medical care.

Her curved spine, combined with hours hunched over her desk to grade papers and all the time she spent carrying her babies on one hip, caused so much pain that she was unable to attend barre classes.

Janice went to two doctors and three specialists seeking relief for her scoliosis. Four of them told her that surgery was the only long-term solution for scoliosis. One doctor recommended placing her in a turtle shell brace to prevent her condition from worsening.

All five of them told her that working out was making things worse, and she needed to stop immediately.

How Janice AVOIDED The Surgery That Doctors Said Was "Inevitable"

Janice didn't have time for surgery—between the busy schedules of her four children, her intense teaching position, waiting around to recover was a luxury she didn't have—and she was absolutely NOT willing to give up her barre classes.

She searched around for other options. Chiropractors helped for a while, but the pain always came back the day after her appointments. Nobody could offer a permanent, natural solution.

Except us.

After only a few weeks of appointments at Berman Physical Therapy, Janice was able to minimize her curve from 30 degrees to 10 degrees through a combination of manual therapy and simple postural exercises. That, combined with a little hip strengthening, was enough to eliminate the back pain within three months.

Not bad, considering the doctors told her recovery was "impossible" without surgery!

Today, nine months after her first appointment, Janice is completely free of low back and hip pain. She is able to maintain her exercise regimen and feels "happier than ever" now that she is "back in control" of her life. She has resumed her normal schedule of four mornings per week at her barre studio, and she has learned to adjust her posture at work so that she no longer slouches over at her desk.

Like most of our athletic patients, Janice is an extremely hard worker. Her dedication and drive helped her get better faster— that's why I love working with athletes! Golfers, swimmers, tennis players, runners…they all see progress quickly in the clinic, because they feel like they have the most to lose if they end up undergoing surgery.

However, when I asked Janice what her biggest worry was about having that scoliosis surgery, she didn't say what I expected to hear. Instead of talking about losing her mobility and having to take a long break from the workout class she loved, she said, "I want to keep being able to bend down and hug my kids. That's the most important thing."

(Feel like your pain is forcing you to miss out on making memories with your family? #6 will change that!)

6. The Inability to Play With Your Grandkids

. . . .

Do you know what about 80% of our clients tell us on their very first phone call with the clinic?

"I can't get on the ground to play with my grandchildren anymore."

"I can't take my granddaughters to the pool."

"I had to miss my grandson's soccer game."

"It feels like I'm missing out on time with my grandkids, but I'm just in too much pain to keep up with them."

There seems to be a trend when it comes to people and pain: they're willing to put up with just about anything until it starts to interfere with the things they love. For some people, that's a sport like golf, tennis, or pickleball. For others, it's relaxing on the beach or traveling to exotic locations.

But I think the final straw for most of the people in my clinic is when their pain takes away the ability to play with their grandkids. Missing out on family time means letting priceless, irreplaceable moments slip by. I've had clients in tears during their first appointments while they tell me about all the big moments they've had to miss in their grandchildren's lives.

One woman, Gretchen, told me about how she fell twice in the hospital as she ran to be present for her granddaughter's birth. "My knees betrayed me," she said. "I knew they were weak. I had been pushing through the pain for years. I had to give up my running, my walks on the beach with my husband, my golfing. But I never thought I'd have to give up family time. I can't believe I missed my own daughter giving birth to her first baby."

Gretchen told me about more events she'd had to miss because of her knee pain: her granddaughter's christening; her grandson's third birthday party (she couldn't handle the long plane ride up north); a family reunion in the Bahamas; a wedding; a dance recital in which two of her grandchildren held starring roles; time in the pool with the four grandkids who came down to Naples for a week over winter vacation; a trip to Disney World with the whole family.

"Pictures and videos aren't the same," Gretchen said tearfully. "I don't want to keep missing these moments. I don't want to be a stranger to my grandkids."

Gretchen told me she felt guilty, too, because every time she skipped a family event, her husband would be forced to stay home and take care of her.

"I tell him to go without me," said Gretchen, "but he always says no. I know it hurts him just as much as it hurts me to look at the pictures and see our grandchildren growing up without us."

Gretchen's story was incredibly moving—and it's not unique! We see people every day whose main motivation for getting better is the desire to spend time with their families.

And because that motivation is so strong—even stronger than the people whose motivation is to get back to playing sports—the people who want to spend more time with their grandchildren are, on average, the ones who get better the fastest.

It took us four months to help Gretchen get her knee pain under control. When she arrived at the clinic for the first time, she couldn't take more than five steps without severe pain. By the time she was discharged, she was walking over a mile per day. After her final appointment, she emailed me pictures of her at the zoo, happily walking between exhibits with her young granddaughter in her arms.

If your aches and pains are forcing you to miss out on family time, you can't afford to waste another day suffering like this. Contact a physical therapist and see what they can do for you.

(#7 is up next, and it's a dizzying one!)

7. Balance

• •

Here are some assumptions we hear ALL THE TIME from people with balance problems:

- *"Balance is something you either have, or you don't."*
- *"The only hope for me is a cane/walker/wheelchair."*
- *"It's an inner ear thing, so I'll need medication or surgery."*

Once you develop a balance problem, your whole world changes.

Where you once felt comfortable and confident, you now start to doubt your abilities.

As your fear of falling grows, your activity level gradually declines, and a few things start to happen.

First, you become less mobile, and by default your strength starts to decline.

Second, you don't get out as much as you used to. Things like going for walks with a spouse, or even just going out and socializing with friends, start to become too much to handle. The emotional impact can be enormous as you start missing out on activities you love in order to protect yourself from a fall.

Now, there is no "one size fits all" diagnosis when it comes to balance. There are three major causes of balance deficiencies: weak muscles, internal ear problems, and neurological conditions.

Luckily, a good physical therapist treats all of them!

The Three Main Causes of Balance Deficiency

1. Weak Muscles

About 80% of our balance-deficient clients have poor balance because of muscle weakness. If you don't have enough strength in the lower half of your body (especially your ankles, quads, hips, and glutes), then you're going to have a hard time maintaining your balance.

How do you gain more strength in these areas? With exercises and workouts! The problem is, people who are unsteady tend to stop exercising altogether. They want to move as little as possible so that they decrease their risk of falling—and the longer they remain inactive, the weaker and less supportive their muscles become! It's a vicious cycle!

2. Inner Ear Problems

As we talked about in the vertigo section, your internal ear consists of a complex canal system. As fluid circulates through the canals, the brain is able to detect where your head is located and help you feel grounded and centered. Here's that picture again:

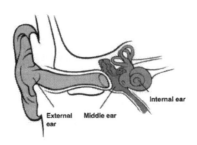

As you age, and you stop a lot of the activities you used to do (like cartwheels and spinning!), the fluid starts having trouble circulating. And when the fluid doesn't circulate, the brain doesn't know where you are, which results in vertigo, dizziness, and a balance deficit!

3. Neurological Conditions

Balance problems are a side effect of all kinds of neurological conditions, including strokes, neuropathy, Parkinson's, and traumatic spinal cord injuries. Conditions like these can interrupt the connection between your brain and your muscles—without that connection, your brain can't tell your muscles when to activate, and so your muscles can't help you remain steady.

Luckily, the brain is smart enough to form new paths to your muscles. Think of it this way: if a major highway, like I-75, shuts down, you can still get to your final destination by taking back roads. A physical therapist is the perfect person to teach you how to find those back roads in your body!

This One Simple Test Can Tell You Everything You Need To Know About Your Balance

If you're not sure which of these three conditions is contributing to your balance problems, there's a simple test you can try right now, in the comfort of your own home! This test will help you see if your balance deficits are muscular—which is the case for 80% of the clients we see.

This will require you to stand on one leg, so make sure you have a helper nearby in case you need to lean on someone quickly!

If you can't stand on one leg, that's okay! Just put one foot directly in front of the other, like you're standing on a tightrope. (Check out the pictures for a visual.)

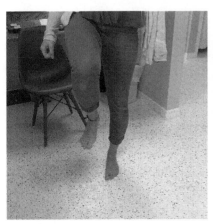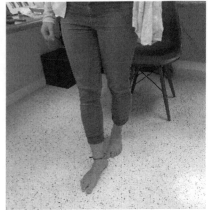

When you're ready, close your eyes and see how long you can balance in that position.

. . . How'd you do?

It was probably MUCH harder with your eyes closed!

DID YOU KNOW: Vision plays a HUGE factor in balance! If you can't see where you are, your brain has a hard time helping you remain steady. This is why a lot of people fall at night—when you get out of bed to use the bathroom or get a drink, the low lighting affects your visibility, and you are more likely to take a tumble.

If you couldn't hold that one-leg stance for more than a few seconds, you're probably relying heavily on your vision for your balance. You might benefit from some strength training!

In the meantime, here are...

The Five Most Common Places People FALL in Their Homes —And The Simple Precautions You Can Take To Make Sure It Doesn't Happen To You Or A Loved One

1. Steps and Stairs

We all know that stairs can be hazardous, so if you have a balance problem, keep all steps in your home free of objects and clutter. Doing this will reduce your chances of tripping! Make sure your stairs are well-lit by having light switches at the top and bottom of the stairs. If your stairs are outdoor, make sure to have a light fitted outside. Automatic motion-sensing lights are the best for that!

2. The Living Room

Make simple changes to your living room, or any area where you spend a lot of time. Take a look at the layout of your furniture. Can you move around easily? Or do you find yourself having to move things out of the way in order to navigate? Move any rugs you might trip over, and make sure any electrical cords are kept neatly tucked away to reduce the risk of falls.

3. The Kitchen

Do you find yourself reaching high to get things out of cabinets and cupboards? Reaching high overhead challenges your balance, and if you have to stand on a chair to get your dishes, you risk a nasty fall! Move items that you use every day down to the lower shelves that you can reach easily.

4. The Bedroom

If you don't have a lamp by your bedside, consider investing in one! When you need to get out of bed (especially in the middle of the night), you need to make sure the area is well-lit—remember how important vision is when it comes to balance! Having a well-lit room will help you move with ease and confidence.

5. The Bathroom

The combination of water and slippery surfaces can be dangerous. Adding non-slip mats (both within and just outside of) your bath and shower will give you extra stability. If you have difficulty getting in and out of the shower or bath, install a "grab bar" so you have something sturdy to grip. Most carpenters can install them quickly near your bath, shower, and toilet!

There you have it! The three most common causes of balance deficits, a very simple test to see how well you're able to balance, and the five most common places within the home that people fall —plus, what you can do to make those places safer for yourself!

If you're ready to stop living in fear of a fall, reach out to a physical therapist and see what options they have for you.

(The 8th condition you didn't realize a PT could help out with is coming next, and it's the one you've been waiting for...)

8. Your Golf Game

• •

If you skipped straight to this section, I have some bad news for you: no amount of physical therapy in the world will make you play like Tiger Woods.

But we can definitely get you closer!

A staggering percentage of our clients tell us they didn't care about their back, neck, knee, or shoulder problem until it started affecting their golf game.

And it makes sense! Most of the people in Naples want to spend their retirements playing golf with their friends—if they're in too much pain to get out on the course, their quality of life starts to diminish.

Then there are the golfers who aren't in any pain at all—they just can't seem to get the scores they want, even after taking lessons with pros or buying expensive clubs.

That's who this section is really for: the people who work with golf pros but aren't improving.

One of our colleagues is a golf pro named Tom. Tom's entire strategy when working with his clients is to teach them how to move their bodies differently. A different grip on the club, a smoother swing, more (or less!) hip rotation...these are all techniques that can massively affect your golf game!

The problem is, *some people physically can't move their bodies the way Tom wants them to.*

Just think about it! A stiff shoulder, elbow, or wrist changes the way you hold the club. A balance deficiency or weight-bearing problem in the knees, hips, or ankles throws off your stance. Limited range of motion in your neck prevents the proper follow-through on your swing.

It can be something so subtle that you have no idea it's happening—but Tom will definitely notice!

Golf Pros Can't Help With This One Important Thing!

Here's where the issues arise:

Even though Tom always figures out where your body position is going wrong, he CAN'T always fix it—or even figure out why it's there in the first place.

A physical therapist can! It's at the core of our very profession —we teach you how to use your body correctly. Once a golf pro like Tom tells you where your physical limitations are, we can help you work on improving them.

We've talked a lot about how your aches and pains are usually symptoms of a bigger problem. Sometimes, that means that the your physical restriction—whether that's in your neck, your shoulder, your back, your hip, your knee, or something else entirely—is actually being caused by a totally different part of your body! It's amazing how often a stiff back is the result of poor posture, or an aching knee can be traced back to weak hips. We even have clients like Scott, from the beginning of this book, who had neck pain that was caused by his broken ankle!

My point is, the root of your problem isn't always obvious.

And golf pros aren't trained to find root problems! They're trained to tell you two things: which techniques you're doing wrong, and what part of your body you need to work on in order to do the techniques right.

They can't tell you HOW to fix that body part, and they can't tell you whether focusing on that body part will solve your root problem...

...which means that if you try to solve the problem on your own, without consulting a physical therapist, you might work for years and never see results!

(That's the case with a HUGE number of our clients!)

So if you're frustrated with your performance out on the course and want to see your golf game improve, start with a pro so you can figure out your limitations...and then head to a physical therapist so you can safely and effectively work through them!

(Exhausted just thinking about all that work? #9 unlocks the secret of how to get a good night's sleep!)

9. Sleeping Better

· ·

We know that the recommended amount of sleep is eight hours per night, but most adults are squeezing by on only five or six!

A good night's sleep in necessary for a healthy lifestyle—from your emotional well-being to your productivity at work to your ability to drive a car without causing an accident. Let's take a quick look at how sleep affects the body:

THE GOOD

A night of good sleep improves…

- Healthy brain function
- Emotional well-being
- Your ability to learn
- Your physical health
- Your body's ability to repair your heart and blood vessels
- Your healthy hormones, like the ones that tell you whether you're hungry and full, and the ones that promote growth
- Your reaction to insulin
- Your immune system
- Your productivity at work or school
- Your muscle mass

THE BAD

A night of poor sleep causes…

- An inability to control your emotions (have you ever seen a toddler melt down when he's tired? That could be you!)
- An increased risk of heart disease
- An increased risk of diabetes, high blood pressure, kidney disease, and stroke
- Less productivity at work or school
- Decreased problem-solving skills
- Lack of focus, memory skills, and driving ability…in fact, driving drowsy is AT LEAST as dangerous as driving while inebriated!

"Okay, okay, I understand what you're saying," you may be thinking. "Sleep is important. The problem is, I can't seem to sleep through the night!"

The problem could be your **sleeping position!** If you ever wake up with a crick in your neck, I can almost guarantee your sleeping position is the culprit.

Why Your Sleeping Position Is (Probably) Harming Your Health

A lot of people who wake up with pain are stomach-sleepers. The WORST thing you can do for your neck is sleep on your stomach—it forces you to turn your head at a 90-degree angle (or else you'll be facedown and suffocate on your pillow!). This position is extremely stressful on the neck, and can even cause strokes. Here's why:

As we age, our cervical spines undergo a degenerative process.

This is completely normal, but it also causes us to lose some of the range of motion that allows our necks to maintain extended positions. Sleeping with the neck extended can, therefore, cause a significant amount of pain, numbness, and tingling! Your body just isn't meant to bend that way. It also causes compression on he blood vessels that deliver blood to your brain, which can cause deadly strokes.

The solution? Try to avoid falling asleep on your stomach. It can be hard to retrain yourself, but your health could depend on it.

Now, if you're NOT a stomach sleeper, you're not off the hook just yet. Pain in back and side sleepers is often related to bedtime, too.

Let me ask you...when's the last time you bought a new pillow?

Side sleepers: You need a thicker pillow to sleep on. It keeps the head and neck in a neutral position. An older pillow won't support your head; it's too compressed from years of use. Just look at the picture below!

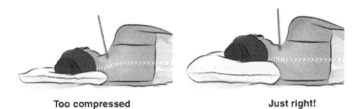

| Too compressed | Just right! |

Back sleepers: a thinner pillow under your head is okay for you—BUT you should still use a thicker pillow under your thighs. Lying in this position will take a lot of stress off your lower back. Make sure the pillow stays under your thighs, NOT your knees.

Side sleepers, you should use three pillows: a thick one under your head, a thick one for under your arm (think of it like you're giving the pillow a hug), and a thick one that goes between your knees. These extra pillows serve to take pressure off the shoulder joints and lower back.

Try out these modifications and see if bedtime improves!

What To Do When Pain ISN'T The Culprit

Now, maybe your lack of sleep isn't related to any pain— maybe you can't get your recommended eight hours because you're just *too stressed to sleep.*

I can't tell you how many clients I see who toss and turn in bed while they worry about the unknown factors of their pain. See if any of these questions resonate with you:

- *"Why can't anyone tell me what's wrong with me?"*
- *"Should I take another pain pill, or will that do more harm than good to my body?"*
- *"How much longer will I have to deal with this pain?"*
- *"How much will it cost to try a different doctor?"*
- *"What if I need surgery?"*
- *"What if it's something really serious, and that's why the doctors can't find an answer?"*
- *"If I keep getting worse, will I have to quit my job?"*
- *"If I quit my job, how will I afford my treatments?"*
- *"How much longer will my insurance pay for my treatments?"*
- *"Why haven't I gotten better yet?"*

- *"What if I never get back to the things I love doing?"*

All of these questions, fears, frustrations, and anxieties can DEFINITELY prevent you from getting the sleep you need—which will only make you feel more frustrated the next morning!

So how can a physical therapist help with this type of stress?

At my clinic, *we answer every single one of those questions at the first appointment.* We make sure you know exactly what is wrong, which techniques we're going to use in order to correct the problem, how many appointments it will take to see improvement, and how much it's all going to cost.

By addressing all of the "unknown" factors and making a solid, specific plan, we destroy all those late-night worries, leaving you feeling relieved and relaxed enough to sleep.

And that good night's sleep will allow your body to focus on repairing itself...which means that you'll wake up in less physical pain, too!

If you have even ONE fear about your pain that's keeping you up at night, finding someone with the answers will make all the difference in the world! Reach out to a physical therapist today—our office is always willing to help out as much as you need us to, both over the phone and in person!

(Most doctors will tell you there's no cure for #10...but they're wrong!)

10. Osteoarthritis

• •

Have you ever heard the term "bone-on-bone?"

A staggering number of clients tell me they have terrible osteoarthritis that has left them "bone-on-bone," and that I'm their last hope before a hip, knee, or shoulder replacement. The truth is that most of the time, the arthritis is completely curable!

What happens is this:

When you go to a doctor to talk about your arthritis, the doctor usually doesn't have time to thoroughly examine you—remember, doctors who accept insurance need to see dozens of patients per day in order to make the clinic profitable! The quickest and easiest solution (for the DOCTOR, not for you!) is to order an X-ray prescribe some pain pills or steroid injections, and, if things look bad in the X-ray, refer you to a surgeon.

But "arthritis" is a huge umbrella term that literally translates to "inflammation of the joint."

And *joint inflammation doesn't need surgery!*

How Terry REVERSED Her Arthritis

Let's talk about symptoms and problems again for a second. Arthritis is only a *symptom.* If you have an inflamed knee, there's something causing that inflammation—it could be the way you stand, or uneven strength in your hips, or any number of other things, but it's not just inflamed *for no reason!* It's the result of something else—a symptom of a different problem.

A great example of an arthritic patient we helped was Terry, a 66-year-old from Marco Island. Terry always noticed pain in her left knee after she played tennis. She went to her doctor, who ordered an X-ray and told her her knee was both "bone-on-bone" and she would need a knee replacement as soon as possible. Terry knew that a surgery that serious would mean the end of her tennis career for the foreseeable future, and so she came to Berman Physical Therapy in a last-ditch effort to buy herself some time before her "inevitable" surgery.

When I sat down with Terry, she told me a key detail that saved her from having her knee replaced: she only had knee pain when she played tennis. There was no pain when she walked—things only flared up on the court.

That detail told me everything I needed to know. Terry's knee wasn't beyond help! She was just doing something wrong when she played tennis. The REAL problem was that her stance on the court was putting extra pressure on her knee, which was irritating the joint and causing the SYMPTOM of arthritis. All we had to do was teach her how to move differently on the tennis court, and we would be able to alleviate the pressure on her knees.

Sure enough, adjusting Terry's stance was enough to take away a significant amount of the inflammation in her knee. With the pressure gone, her body began to heal itself, and she avoided having a knee replacement.

Terry's situation is an extremely common one we see in the clinic—but we also see people who are much worse off, because they have let their arthritis stop them from moving altogether! When a joint becomes inflamed, it can be extremely painful to move. But the longer you go without moving, the stiffer you're going to become—which means that movement becomes even MORE painful!

How John Undid 40 YEARS' Worth Of Damage

I'll give you an example of a client whose arthritis was much more difficult to cure than Terry's. John is a 72-year-old from Estero, and when I met him, he had such intense inflammation in his knuckles that he couldn't open his hand. John's son, Louis, called us up and asked if we'd ever seen anything like that before (we had) and whether we'd be able to help (we could!).

Louis brought John in for his first appointment and even took notes as I explained to John that the only way to alleviate the pain in his hand was to get the joints moving again.

After only one appointment, I had helped John open his hand enough to hold a tennis ball. I told him to hold onto that tennis ball and practice gently squeezing it at least ten times per day until our next meeting. He and Louis were filled with excitement as they left the office—after four decades of searching, they had finally found a doctor who could improve John's arthritis!

But when our next meeting rolled around…John was even WORSE than before!

"I don't know what happened," Louis told me. "I call him every day to ask if he's been doing his exercises, and he always says yes."

But John told a different story. When I asked him if he was doing his homework, he shrugged. "It was too hard," he said. "I couldn't do it."

That's what happens with people who don't work on improving their arthritis! It gets worse and worse, until even something as simple as *holding a tennis ball* is too painful.

We worked again on getting John's fingers to spread, but I could tell he was resistant. No matter how much Louis and I encouraged him, he was convinced that the manual therapy I was administering was a waste of time.

Slowly, I realized what the problem was...

John didn't *want* to get better!

Or rather, he DID want to get better, but he was hoping for a "miracle cure" that would get his hand back to normal immediately, without any hard work on his part.

That's never the case with physical therapy. If it took decades for John's hand to become so inflamed, it was going to take at *least* a few weeks of solid effort to get everything moving again.

Once John understood that there was no "quick fix" for his pain, he started making much better progress. We took things a little at a time, and before long he was opening and closing his hand without a problem!

If you suffer from osteoarthritis and fear that there's no cure, *never* rule out physical therapy! A good clinic will be able to help you out, so reach out before your situation gets any worse!

Chapter Five:

Retraining Your Brain

• •

This is the end of PART I: A PARADIGM SHIFT.

Hopefully you have a good understanding of my clinic's mission: to treat problems, not symptoms, and to teach people like you that it's important to take the whole person into consideration instead of just focusing on "where it hurts." As I learned from Jenni's gluten allergy, when we zoom in too closely, we miss things—important things—that can completely change diagnoses, treatment plans, and lives.

It takes a lot of "brain retraining" to think this way. We're so immersed in western medicine ideas about insurance companies knowing what's best for us. We treat pain pills and surgeries as if they're cures, and we ignore how dangerous, expensive, and ultimately futile those solutions can be. We refuse to look at "the rest" and choose to focus only on what MRIs, X-rays, and blood tests say about our bodies.

And for the sake of our health, *we need to stop.*

By reading PART I of this book, you have taken the first step toward retraining your brain.

In PART II: HEAD TO TOE, I'll go into specific details about each part of the body and explain some of the science behind why that part of the body might hurt. I'll also give you tips and tricks you can use right now, in the comfort of your own home, to start feeling better. This part of the book is not linear—you can skip the chapters that don't apply to you, but I highly recommend reading them all. You know now that pain in one area can be caused by a problem in another, and you will get a much clearer picture of how the body parts work together if you read every chapter!

PART II

Head To Toe

Chapter Six:

Neck

• •

Take a moment and write down ten things you do on your computer, tablet, or phone every day. Don't read the next page until you've filled in all ten!

1. _____

2. _____

3. _____

4. _____

5. _____

6. _____

7. _____

8. _____

9. _____

10. _____

Here's my list:

1. Check social media
2. Text/call/video chat with friends and family
3. Shop online (Amazon is my weakness!)
4. Read articles or e-books
5. Use my GPS
6. Update my calendar
7. Send emails
8. Take photos and videos
9. Organize my finances
10. "Fun" stuff, like playing games or watching Netflix

My list was easy. I came up with it in less than a minute, and if I hadn't been limited to ten items, I probably could have kept going.

Technology has completely changed the way we live our lives. In many ways, it's a huge convenience (like I said, Amazon is a godsend). But in other ways, the ubiquity of technology is extremely detrimental. It's taking a toll on your body, even if you think you're not spending "that much" time hunched over a screen!

You see, over the past decade—or, more accurately, since the introduction of the smartphone—studies have shown that humans are spending drastically more time sitting than ever. It's had such a huge impact that we as a nation are now spending more money treating the adverse effects of sitting than we are spending on the adverse effects of smoking.

Look back at your list.

Think about where you are when you're doing those things on your phone, tablet, or computer. What does your body look like? What kind of posture do you have? Are you sitting? Lying down? Hunched over?

If you're reading this in a public place, glance around. Notice how many people are looking at their electronic devices. Study the way their necks crane down toward their screens, the way their chins jut out, the way their shoulders slump forward.

Or, if you're not in a public place, pay attention the next time you go out somewhere. When you're in the car at a red light, look to your left and right. At least one of those people will be looking down at their phone—and it is highly unlikely that they are looking for directions to where they are going.

Your Phone Is Ruining Your Neck—And Here's The Scientific Proof

All this "screen time" has dramatically increased the prevalence of neck pain.

Ten years ago, the majority of the people with neck pain were older (at least 65) and most likely worked at a desk job their entire lives.

It was rare to see neck pain in someone younger, unless it was related to a traumatic incident like a car crash.

Nowadays, the majority of the neck pain I treat is in people *under* 65.

So why does all this "screen time" create neck pain?

Take a look at this picture—I have a copy of it framed in my office:

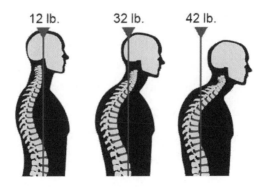

12 lb.   32 lb.   42 lb.

That picture is the perfect example of "text neck." Text neck is a form of poor posture—basically, it's a popular new buzzword for an overuse syndrome that affects the necks of frequent phone users. In that picture, you can see the way your posture affects the forces placed on your neck and spine. With normal, "proper" posture, the average head weighs around 12 pounds. For every inch you let your head fall forward, you dramatically increase the force placed on your spine, and therefore the head starts to feel heavier and heavier.

Think of your spine like a stack of building blocks you played with as a kid.

If you build your tower straight up, whatever you place on top will have a very sturdy foundation. It will be completely supported by the blocks under it, and the forces of gravity won't be able to topple it over. This is what happens with proper posture: the spine supports the head.

Now, when you take your head *out* of alignment, like the second and third figures in our picture, the force of gravity becomes much more of a problem.

It would be like trying to attach a bowling ball to the side of your tower with Scotch tape; the set-up is unstable and the bowling ball is too heavy, so the whole thing falls apart.

Of course, your spine is much stronger than some building blocks, so you're not going to crumple to the floor in pieces like our metaphorical tower.

Instead, you're going to make your body work much harder to keep your head from falling off. The longer the poor posture goes on, the more overworked the muscles, tendons, and ligaments in your neck will become. In time, they will become strained, exhausted, and chronically weak. The muscles at the base of your skull will eventually become ischemic (lacking blood flow). All of this adds up to headaches and neck pain, but it's only half the equation.

Look around you again, if you're in a public place. 99% of the people looking at their phones are probably holding it at, or just above, waist height. In order to hold something at this height and in this position, you have to roll your shoulders forward and round your upper back.

Holding this position for an extended amount of time takes a severe toll on your body; it lengthens your scapular retractors (those are the muscles between your shoulder blades and spine), which ends up weakening those muscles over time. From there, it's a vicious cycle—the weak muscles lead to worse posture, which lengthens the muscles even more, which weakens them, which leads to worse posture....

It's like there's no escape!

Margaret's Doctor Wanted Her to Stay On Pills—She Had Other Ideas

One client who got caught in the vicious cycle was Margaret, a 67-year-old woman from Naples.

When I first got a call from Margaret, she told me that she had had progressively worsening neck pain for the past year-and-a-half. At the time, she was 66, and had recently retired from her lifelong job working at a bank. She had occasionally played golf on the weekends while in the workforce, but after retirement she increased to playing three or four times a week.

Margaret remembers her neck being a little stiff and sore when she was working, but everything always "worked itself out" with some over-the-counter pain medicine. But about a year ago, she developed a pain in her neck that just wouldn't go away!

She tried everything she could think of: decreasing her time on the golf course, putting heating pads on her neck in the mornings and evenings, going for massages...nothing worked!

After about three months of pain, Margaret made an appointment with her doctor. He wrote her a prescription for pain medicine and took an X-ray. The X-ray showed mild degenerative changes—totally normal for someone her age—but nothing to explain her constant neck pain.

Her doctor was at a loss. He told her to try the pain meds and come back in a month if she wasn't feeling better.

Now, pain meds, as I've discussed over and over again in this book and in my clinic, are not a real cure. They mask the pain, and they might make you feel better for a little while, but as soon as they wear off, you're right back where you started. Actually, you're WORSE than when you started, because those pain pills are slowly and quietly damaging your internal organs. Plus, you get more and more frustrated with each pill, because you know they're only buying you temporary relief!

Pain is a symptom of something bigger; and if you only treat the symptoms, your problem will NEVER go away.

Needless to say, Margaret didn't get better using pain medication. One month later, when she arrived at her follow-up appointment, her doctor did two things:

1) He refilled her prescription (which Margaret knew wouldn't help!)

2) He referred her to an orthopedic surgeon for a consultation

After waiting FIVE WEEKS for an opening to get in to see the surgeon, Margaret was told that she needed an MRI before the surgeon could be sure that surgery was the best option. The MRI showed the exact same results as the X-ray: mild degeneration (again, this is normal for anyone Margaret's age) but nothing "surgical."

The orthopedic surgeon referred Margaret to a physical therapy practice that he owned. She went three times per week for six weeks, but there was still no improvement.

When I asked her what kind of treatment they were providing at that physical therapy clinic, this is what she told me:

"They gave me a sheet with my stretches and exercises on it. I'd go do them by myself, or sometimes with a tech, and then they'd put some ice and a TENS unit on me at the end. That was pretty much it."

This is a very common response, and one that we discussed over and over in Part I of this book! Physical therapy clinics that operate in-network aren't able to give you their full attention; they're running around trying to get to four patients per hour, which means that for the majority of your appointment, you're stuck on your own, or with an assistant who knows nothing about your particular problem.

Does that sound like a recipe for success? It sure wasn't for Margaret! She reported no lasting improvement after every single appointment.

After six weeks of failed PT, the surgeon recommended cortisone injections to help with the pain. Luckily, this is where Margaret put her foot down—she had heard horror stories from her friends on the golf course about how painful this type of injection could be, and she also knew that having even MORE pain medicine was not the long-term solution she was seeking for her neck.

Margaret found my clinic by doing a quick Google search and reading some online reviews of Berman Physical Therapy. The top review at the time was from a someone with neck pain—someone we had cured in just a few weeks, without any medication. Margaret knew she had finally found her answer.

She called us and booked a session, where we spent time going over her full history (including her job at the bank, her love of golf, and the hobbies she couldn't do anymore now that the neck pain was so bad) and checking out her neck.

What Was ACTUALLY Wrong With Margaret

I determined pretty quickly that Margaret's neck pain was the result of poor posture. She had leaned over her desk to look at paperwork all those years at the bank, and the tiny print on the forms she needed to fill out had forced her to crane her neck down in order to see.

It's exactly the same position a lot of office workers use as they squint at their computer screens.

(It could be exactly the same position you use every day to text!)

Like we talked about earlier in this chapter, maintaining this position for an extended amount of time takes a severe toll on your body. Think about that picture again:

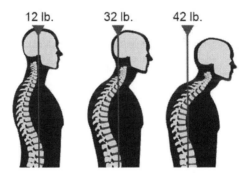

Margaret looked like the person on the right. All that "hunching" over the years had stretched out the muscles between her shoulder blades and spine, which made them weak, so she couldn't hold her neck up properly.

For Margaret to correct her posture on her own would be like someone who has never been to the gym trying to bench-press 200 pounds—impossible without a lot of strength training! The muscles Margaret needed were just too weak.

And here's where the vicious cycle kicks in. See if you can follow this:

The more Margaret leaned over into a poor posture position, the heavier her head became (check that picture again!).

The heavier her head became, the harder her muscles had to work, and the farther they stretched.

The farther her muscles stretched, the weaker they became.

The weaker the muscles became, the harder it was for Margaret to use proper posture.

And the more Margaret used IM-proper posture, the heavier her head became...

...so her muscles worked harder and stretched farther...

...so they became weaker...

...so proper posture became harder...

...so Margaret used improper posture...

...so her head got heavier...

You get the point!

Repeat that cycle every day for years, and you've got a sure recipe for neck pain!

The ONLY Way To Cure Neck Pain Like Margaret's

After Margaret's first appointment at my clinic, I asked her how she felt.

She rolled her neck around a little. "Amazing. I feel amazing!"

Isn't that crazy!? Margaret had spent six months going through X-rays, MRIs, two refills of pain medication, and 18 sessions of physical therapy at the other clinic...and all it took was one session of manual therapy with someone who wanted to figure out the underlying cause of her pain for her to feel "amazing!"

Manual therapy—the only type of physical therapy that we do at my clinic—works like a really intense massage. I figure out which muscles are causing pain, and then I use special hands-on techniques on those muscles to loosen and strengthen them. In Margaret's case, the muscles that needed attention were the ones down between her shoulder blades, which were exhausted and irritated from struggling to hold up her head.

But the real magic happens after the manual therapy, when the muscles are finally loosened up and the joints are moving better. This is the part where we retrain your muscles—if I were to skip that part, Margaret's neck would fall right back into the position she was used to, and she would wind up in pain again. That's why massage therapy had never helped her; she felt great after the massage, but she couldn't maintain proper posture (she didn't even know there was a problem with her posture!) and so she constantly "undid" all the progress she had made in her massages by putting stress on her muscles all over again.

Retraining your muscles can be very difficult. That's because it's not just about your muscles—you also have to retrain your brain!

Think of it this way: if you're right-handed, you can sign your name using your right hand without even thinking about it. But if I asked you to sign your name with your LEFT hand, it's going to be much more challenging.

Why is that? Both hands use exactly the same muscles, joints, tendons, and ligaments. It should be easy!

The problem is, your brain has no idea how to control all the soft tissues in your left hand! It would take a lot of training (remember how long it took you to learn to write back in elementary school?) to get your left-handed signature to look as good as your right-handed signature.

That is essentially what the other physical therapist was asking Margaret to do at her first clinic: use muscles that had never been trained. Handing her a sheet of paper with stretches and exercises to do on her own, without EVER teaching her how to do them or training her brain to control her muscles in a new way, had NO CHANCE of working out.

During one of my earliest sessions with Margaret, I put my hands on her shoulder blades and pulled her back into the exact posture I wanted her to use.

"Now you know what it feels like to stand correctly," I said. "Do you feel which muscles are activated and which aren't?"

She said she did—and she was surprised by how different it felt to stand correctly!

By physically putting Margaret into the right position, I was doing two things: showing her muscles where they needed to be, and allowing her brain to memorize which muscles needed to "turn on" in order to achieve this posture. It set her up for success.

We spent the whole session—and the next one—working on finding that posture. The first few times, she needed my help. But soon, she was able to find the right position on her own.

She started golfing again. She stopped taking pain pills. She slept through the night.

Eventually, she stopped needing physical therapy appointments.

It took, from start to finish, four weeks at my clinic.

Do You Have Posture Like Margaret's? Here's A Quick Test!

If you have neck pain and noticed any similarities to Margaret's struggle, here's a quick test that will let you evaluate your posture.

(Side note: Margaret's pain happened slowly and gradually over a period of years. There are other forms of neck pain that come on more quickly: neck pain caused by traumatic events, like car crashes, can STILL be related to posture if it lingers more than a few months! Try a physical therapist before a surgeon.)

Here's the posture test:

Find a flat, empty wall.

Stand up as tall as possible and press your heels against the wall, keeping your feet flat on the floor.

Now press the rest of your body against the wall, starting from the bottom up. Focus on your calves, your glutes, your upper back, and your head.

Stand in this position and feel how much your back is arched, how much your neck needs to bend backwards in order for your head to reach the wall. Try to picture what your body looks like to a bystander.

Have someone take a picture of you from the side so you can

compare your mental image of yourself to a real image. If you have a significant arch in your back or bend in your neck—or if it was impossible for you to get into the position I'm describing—you probably have poor posture. This could explain any neck pain you may have.

Fortunately, there are ways to retrain your brain and muscles to improve your posture and eliminate this pain. Even if you don't have neck pain at this time, poor posture will, more likely that not, lead to discomfort in the future, so it's best to act preemptively. Find your nearest manual physical therapy clinic and set up a consultation today.

Skip ahead to the BONUS chapter at the end of this book for links to more absolutely free resources you can utilize to help you out with your neck pain.

Chapter Seven:

Elbow

• •

You know, the funny thing about "tennis elbow" is that you can get it without ever picking up a racket in your life!

(That's what we're going to focus on for this chapter: lateral epicondylitis, AKA tennis elbow, which is the most common elbow-related issue we see in the clinic.)

Tennis elbow occurs when the tendons in your elbow get overloaded and inflamed. It usually happens after a lot of repetitive motions—like swinging a tennis racket! Check out this picture for a visual:

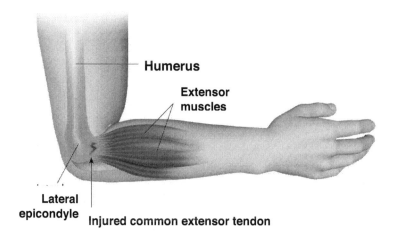

If you've ever had tennis elbow, you know that it can be

excruciating. I once had a client tell me his arm was so sensitive that "you can't even touch it with a cotton ball!"

There is a huge industry geared toward tennis elbow treatment. You may have seen a tennis elbow brace or strap, which wraps around your forearm and applies very tight compression to the wrist extensor muscles. This type of solution is a lot like the theory of "when you bang your leg on something, start rubbing it to make it feel better." Technically, you're not doing anything, but the sensation of rubbing your leg desensitizes the area and sends a different kind of feedback to the brain, which takes your attention away from the pain. A tennis elbow brace takes your attention away from the pain, but it does nothing to actually cure you! Just like pain medications, it's a "mask" instead of a treatment.

Speaking of pain medications, I've seen dozens of "magic creams" that claim to provide relief for tennis elbow. Again, these are just masks. The cream may feel great when it first hits your skin, but eventually the sensation wears off, and you're right back where you started. I've seen people try this type of treatment for YEARS. They spend *hundreds or thousands of dollars* on their preferred cream, which they have to reapply every few hours, and they come to depend on it in order to function! That's not a real solution, either.

A lot of people decide to seek help from an orthopedic specialist. That prompts the usual routine of X-rays, MRIs, cortisone injections, and possibly surgery. I have yet to meet anyone who has tried these techniques and found 100% relief—including surgery!

Tennis Elbow Is Secretly The EASIEST Thing To Fix

I love treating tennis elbow. It's one of the simplest things to fix—and it AMAZES people when they see how I do it!

(We're going to dive into a little bit of science and anatomy for this section. I'll try to keep it as easy as I can, but if you ever get confused, it might benefit you to Google a picture or two so you can visualize what I'm talking about.)

A few years ago, I had a client named Harvey who came to the clinic with tennis elbow. He played in a tennis league with other people aged 60+, and his doubles partner was counting on him for an upcoming tournament.

Harvey had already tried all the braces and creams he could find and had had no luck. His doctor told him that the next step was surgery, but Harvey wasn't willing to use that option so close to the tournament. He knew he'd never recover in time.

At Harvey's first appointment with me, I didn't even touch his elbow. I poked around it and made sure it bent, extended, and rotated the way it was supposed to, but I didn't give it any treatment. Still, Harvey reported a 50% improvement in his pain level by the end of the session!

How is that possible if I never worked on his elbow?

Could it be because the elbow is a *symptom* of a problem that is *somewhere else*?

YES! Would you believe me if I said that the neck is the most common cause of elbow pain?

(Here's where things get a little science-y.) Earlier, we said that tennis elbow is just another name for lateral epicondylitis: your wrist extensors (AKA the muscles that extend your wrist) are attached to the lateral epicondyle, which is a round protuberance on your elbow bone. The lateral epicondyle forms a joint—it's what lets you bend and unbend your elbow! Check out the picture:

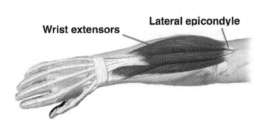

Wrist extensors   Lateral epicondyle

When those wrist extensors become inflamed and swollen, they cause pain. Now, there is a very important nerve called the *radial nerve* that gets involved with your wrist extensors:

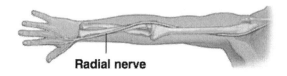

Radial nerve

The radial nerve supplies power and feeling to the wrist extensors. It also originates from the neck.

Let's take a look at the neck. When a nerve comes out of your spinal column, it forms what is called a "nerve root." Several nerve roots combine with each other to create nerves, which travel away from the spine and affect whatever part of the body they're supposed to affect. In the case of the radial nerve shown above, that part of the body is the arm, including the wrist extensors.

If you trace the radial nerve all the way back to its root in the spinal column, you'll discover that it leads to the bottom of your cervical spine, which is the lower half of your neck.

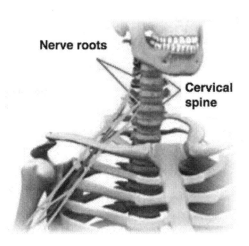

Nerve roots

Cervical spine

This means that the nerve roots that begin in your neck are the power source for your wrist extensors. In other words, pain in your wrist extensors (and the elbow they're attached to) can be caused by problems in your neck!

To demonstrate what kinds of problems I'm talking about, I'm going to give you an analogy. Picture a garden hose, like the kind you might use to water your plants. The water is flowing freely... but what happens if you step on the hose? The water will still come out, but it will be much more strained—a very weak trickle instead of a stream.

The same thing can happen to the nerve roots in your cervical spine!

When you extend your neck (as if you're looking up at the

stars), the position compresses the vertebrae in your spinal column, which presses down on the nerve roots the same way your foot pressed down on the hose.

Nerves are EXTREMELY temperamental! They do not like being pressed, and even the most minimal stress on a nerve root can cause a flare up. This can result in anything from numbness to a dull ache to, in extreme cases, hypersensitivity ("You can't even touch my elbow with a cotton ball!"). Just like the garden hose, any kind of compression on a nerve root will affect how everything flows.

"But I don't walk around with my neck craned back to look at the sky all day long," you might be thinking. "How does this nerve root theory explain my elbow pain!?"

Because it doesn't have to be the sky you're staring at all day.

If you read the neck pain chapter right before this one, you already know what I'm talking about: technology.

Nowadays, almost everyone has some kind of electronic device that they use every day, whether that's a smartphone, a tablet, a laptop, or a desktop computer. If you're reading this book in a public place, look around you—I bet at *least* half of the people you see are using some kind of technology, and I bet their posture looks something like this:

- Shoulders hunched forward
- Neck craning down toward the screen
- Chin jutted out
- If there's a phone involved, the phone is held at or just above waist height

This position is very hard on your neck! Even though you

aren't tipping your head back, you're still putting pressure on those nerve roots because of the way your chin is positioned. The farther forward your chin goes, the more extended your neck will be.

Check the picture to see what I mean:

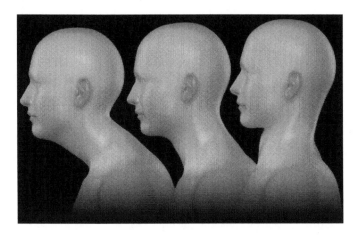

In the model on the far left, you can clearly see rounded shoulders and a very sharp angle where the back of the head meets the neck—and you can imagine all the nerve roots being crunched and causing pain all over the body!

It can even cause pain in…you guessed it…the elbow.

It probably won't surprise you to learn that my client, Harvey, had a career that required him to sit and stare at a screen for most of the day. He worked in human resources, and although he tried to stay active after work, he still practiced poor posture at his desk for eight hours every day.

After going through some very basic postural changes, Harvey reported that his tennis elbow was 50% better—and I never even touched his elbow! All I did was move his neck into a position that didn't compress any nerve roots, and most of the pain immediately disappeared. After a few sessions of physical therapy and doing his homework, he was back on the tennis court.

Time To Take Action!

If your elbow hurts, or if you sit longer than you stand on an average day, try this out.

Find a large wall and put your back against it, keeping your feet about 6 inches away from the wall. Your knees should be slightly bent and "soft."

Now, keep your tailbone, upper back, and the back of your head against the wall at the same time...WITHOUT extending your neck!

Hold that position and slowly try to make the back of your neck touch the wall.

Chances are, as you try to push the back of your neck against the wall, your low back will start to arch, but don't let it. Keep your knees soft and try to press both the small of your back and the back of your neck against that wall.

(It's impossible, by the way, so don't hurt yourself! Just get as close as you can.)

Feel what that position does to your chin. It should be pulled down and in, almost like you're creating a "double chin."

What you're doing here is putting the neck into *flexion* (the opposite of extension)! Doing this helps to release those compressed nerve roots, which will alleviate the pain.

Maintaining this position on the wall may be extremely difficult, especially for people with elbow pain, but if you can hold it for at least 30 seconds and practice every hour, on the hour, you'll start seeing results very quickly!

Skip ahead to the BONUS chapter at the end of this book for links to more absolutely free resources you can utilize to help you out with your elbow pain.

Chapter Eight:

Back

. . . .

If you're familiar with the Naples area, you know that golf courses around here are far from scarce. With nearly 100 courses, it's no surprise that we attract golfers (especially retired ones) from around the world…and it's also no surprise that quite a few of them suffer from back pain.

Now, I would never put myself in a "box" by saying that I only treat golfers with back pain, but because of the area where my clinic is located, at least 75% of the clients we see are just that: golfers with back pain! It's given me a lot of practice, and so back pain has become one of my specialties.

But back pain is also something I've been through myself. I had just graduated from PT school when I injured my back. It happened at the gym—I was always pushing myself to get stronger, and that day, I added more weight to the bar than I had ever lifted before.

As I lifted the bar, I remember feeling something in my lower back that just didn't feel right. I pushed through the pain and finished my workout, but later that night, my back was really bothering me.

The next morning, I could barely get out of bed! There was a very strange pain shooting down my left leg—a telltale sign of a herniated disc.

Luckily, I worked at a physical therapy clinic!

This was before I had started Berman Physical Therapy, but I still had access to people who knew how to fix my back pain...or so I thought.

My boss worked on my back at least twice a day, and I did my exercises every chance I got. Within two weeks, I was 90% better —but I just couldn't clear that last 10%!

Slowly, I got back to my normal routine. I was back at the gym, although I was worried that lifting would injure me further, so I never worked out as aggressively as I wanted to. I found myself limiting my movements, just in case something caused my back to flare up. No matter what I was doing, I always felt a slight discomfort in my lower back—only on the left, but always present.

I fell into a vicious cycle: the less I moved, the worse my pain became. Driving made my back stiffen up; sitting on the couch for longer than 30 minutes was unbearable. Stretching helped, but not for long, and never enough to get me back to feeling 100%.

It wasn't until a year and a half later, when I moved to Jacksonville, that I finally found the cure. That was where I met Aaron Robles, a physical therapist who specializes in functional manual therapy (the main focus of my own PT practice today!). Aaron hired me to work for his practice, and through his mentorship, I learned that the key to healing pain is treating problems, not symptoms. Aaron never focused on what was hurting—he wanted to figure out *why* it was hurting.

Learning Aaron's methods completely changed how I handled

my own back pain. I asked him to take a look at my left lower back, but he insisted on assessing my entire body. At the end of his evaluation, he had figured out that the problem was actually on my *right* side! My right side was weaker than my left, he said, and so I was compensating by overworking the left side. He explained that by strengthening my right side, I would be able to eliminate the pain on my left.

It sounded crazy.

I did what he told me to do anyway.

Three months later, I was about two hours into a road trip from Naples to Jacksonville when I turned around to reach for something in the backseat—and realized that my back didn't hurt.

I wiggled around in my seat a little bit more to see if I'd been imagining it, but it was real! For the first time in almost two years, I was 100% pain-free.

My Back Pain Story Could Be YOUR Back Pain Story!

The majority of the clients we see at Berman Physical Therapy have a back pain story very similar to my own. Sometimes they injured it in a very specific event, like lifting something too heavy. Sometimes the pain started after something ridiculous, like an extra-hard sneeze. And sometimes it's just been there for years, gradually getting worse and worse.

But one thing's for sure: the more people "rest" to help their back pain heal, the worse they get!

This may go against every instinct you have, but "taking it easy" is one of the *worst* things you can do for back pain. I remember restricting my movement and limiting my workouts after my herniated disc because I was so afraid of putting myself through more pain, but that just caused more complications, and made my recovery ten times longer.

Here's why movement is so important for healing low back pain:

Every time you move, you activate your muscles.

Muscle activation increases blood flow.

Increased blood flow brings brings fresh nutrients to the areas within your body that need them the most—for example, the injury site in your back!

What happens if you DON'T move around very much after a back injury?

Well, for starters, you won't be using your muscles as often as you should. That means your blood flow is going to be significantly reduced, which in turn reduces the fresh nutrients to the area that is injured. This means that the injured area can't heal efficiently, and the likelihood that it will be re-injured will be high.

(Isn't it ironic that the very thing you're doing to prevent re-injury is actually making your back more susceptible to re-injury!?)

People eventually realize that rest isn't helping to alleviate their back pain, and so they start reaching for the over-the-counter pain medication. We've talked before about how pain medications just "mask" the pain and don't actually help you heal—in a lot of cases, they give you a false sense of relief. Because you're (temporarily) out of pain, you end up pushing your body to do things that the pain would normally prevent you from doing...and then, when the medication wears off, you feel all the pain catch up with you again!

"Wait a second…I've had back pain before that healed up after some medication," you might be thinking. And that's entirely possible! Once the medication has taken the edge off the pain and you feel comfortable moving again, you jumpstart that process we talked about earlier: your muscle contractions cause an increase in blood flow, which delivers much-needed nutrients to the areas that need to heal.

But it's not always that simple. Some people get stuck for years, or even decades—they just don't move enough to heal the area. And, as we've talked about before, the less someone moves, the stiffer they get, and the more painful motion becomes…so the less they move…and the stiffer they get…until they reach the point where even something as minimal as picking up a pencil or sneezing is enough to throw them into unbearable agony.

Finally, after the pain becomes too much to bear, people who have been caught up in the vicious back pain cycle reach for the phone and call their doctor. The doctor will prescribe a medication: "Take this for a month and come back if it doesn't get better!"

Of course, it doesn't get better. The masking effect of the pain pills won't help at this stage of the game—by now, years have gone by, and the injured back is so stiff and weak from lack of use that something as simple as "moving around" won't be enough to fix the problem!

So the patient ends up back at the doctor. The doctor writes another prescription for more pills, and also takes an X-ray. The X-ray shows mild degeneration—all very normal, especially in people over age 50—but doesn't find anything conclusive that's causing the pain.

The next step might be an MRI, or a visit to an orthopedic surgeon, or a trip to a specialist for some injections and epidurals. Ultimately, though, back pain sufferers tend to wind up in the same place: physical therapy.

(Wouldn't it be great if you could have skipped all those other steps and come here first!?)

Now, as we've talked about before in this book, most physical therapy clinics in town are in-network and productivity-driven. That means that the physical therapist will see 3–4 patients per hour, so that they can bill insurance companies for as much reimbursement as possible and keep the clinic profitable. Spending 15 minutes with a patient is not enough time to provide quality treatments, of course—the PT barely has time to ask what part of you hurts, much less figure out what underlying problems are *actually* causing your symptoms!

It's also physically impossible to give someone quality manual therapy in only 15 minutes. In order to perform manual therapy effectively, the physical therapist must constantly assess and reassess the patient...but there's barely even time for the *first* assessment!

So what happens to your back?

Short answer: it doesn't get better.

Long answer: you do some stretches and exercises as outlined on a piece of paper that the physical therapist hands you. You might have a technician in the room to watch you or help you out, but you'll never really know if you're doing the exercises correctly, and you'll never push yourself through pain—at least, not hard enough for it to make a difference. You'll get some electric stim to promote blood flow (not as effective as moving your muscles) and you'll get some ice for your back (couldn't you be doing this at home, without the commute and the copay!?) and you'll probably have to come back three times per week until the insurance allotment runs out.

But that's not the worst part...

The WORST part is that the patients who go through this now think that they have "tried everything."

So what do they do? They head back to the doctor! They tell the doctor that nothing has helped, that they're out of options, and they *ask for surgery.*

Sometimes, they get what they ask for, but other times surgeons will refuse to operate—yet. They take a few more X-rays and MRIS and determine that there's nothing warranting surgery, so the patient should just "deal with the pain" until things get bad enough for an invasive procedure to be justified.

Just "deal with it!"

Just *wait for it to get worse!*

Just keep taking these horrible pain pills and half-heartedly practicing the physical therapy exercises that have never helped, and wait until the inevitable surgery date!

It is usually around this time when people realize there has to be another way. They turn to Google, or they start asking their friends, and eventually, the lucky ones stumble upon my clinic.

By the time people call me, they are very hesitant to commit to physical therapy again. All they know about physical therapy is the experience that we just talked about.

"I've already tried physical therapy and it didn't work. How are you any different?"

You already know how we're different: we treat problems, not symptoms, in order to help people aged 50+ keep active and free of pain meds...even when their doctors and kids are telling them to "just take it easy!"

How I Gave Dolores Her Life Back

A client of mine named Dolores went through everything I outlined above, from the pills to the physical therapy to the "deal with it and wait for surgery" advice.

When Dolores called me, she had been suffering from back pain for over 50 years. At age 68, that was the majority of her life! She had injured her back while running on the track team in high school, and her coach had advised her to take a break from the team and rest until it felt better—but it never did.

Dolores was so afraid of re-injuring her back that she quit running altogether. She became less and less active, and yet her back hurt more and more! She told me the pain had always been on the left side of her low back (just like mine after my herniated disc!), but that her X-rays and MRIs showed that everything was completely normal.

I ran a few tests at Dolores's first appointment that told me everything I needed to know.

For the entire first session, I didn't touch Dolores's back, or anything on the left side of her body. Instead, I worked on her *right* hip. Just like with my own back troubles, Dolores's right side was weaker than her left. She was compensating by overworking the left side. By strengthening her right side, she would be able to eliminate the pain on her left.

Using manual techniques that the "cookie cutter" physical therapist hadn't had time to perform, I improved Dolores's right hip mobility, which took an enormous amount of pressure off her left side. Dolores's joints were very stiff from all those years of limiting her motion; as soon as I helped her loosen up and get moving again, the blood flow and nutrients increased, and she felt the effects immediately.

"I can't believe how good I feel already," Dolores told me after our first session. "I thought I was out of options."

I gave Dolores three exercises to work on at home to make sure she kept moving before our next appointment, and by the time she came back, she had made a huge leap of improvement!

Dolores ended up needing to come in for about twelve sessions —that's a VERY small number, considering how many years she had been in pain!

She didn't go back to the surgeon, and she's off all pain medication for the first time since high school.

All it took was addressing her problem, instead of her symptoms, and getting her moving again.

The Test I Gave Dolores—That You Can Try RIGHT NOW

If you are over age 50 and have some type of desk job (or if you spend more time sitting than standing in your day-to-day life), this will save your back. It's the same test I gave Dolores!

Sit in a firm chair and keep your back nice and tall. Take your right leg and cross it over your left in a way that leaves your right ankle on top of your left knee. Check the picture for a visual:

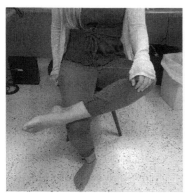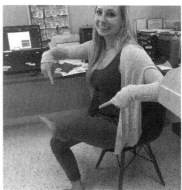

Take note of the stretch you may be feeling in your right hip area. Don't try to force your knee down toward the floor; just let it rest comfortably. Notice its position, and keep it in mind for later —it may help to have someone take a picture of you, or to use a mirror.

Now switch legs! Do the same exact thing, but this time place your left ankle on your right knee. Does this side feel looser or tighter than the first side? Does your left knee drop lower than your right knee did, or is it higher?

Chances are, there is at least a slight discrepancy between the sides. Whichever side feels tighter—that is, whichever side had the higher knee—is the side we need to work on.

You can work on loosening this hip right now, in the comfort of your own home! Here's how:

Stand in front of the kitchen sink. Grab onto the countertop for balance. Now, keeping both knees straight, pick one foot straight up off the ground without letting your foot swing forward or side-to-side. Don't let those knees bend! The motion should be coming from your pelvis, not from your legs.

If you feel at all unsteady, don't proceed with this test without a reliable helper there to spot you!

Now, as you balance on one foot, slowly release your grip on the counter and see how long you can stand there without using your hands. Maybe it's a few seconds; maybe it's closer to a minute! Maybe you can't do it at all. That's okay!

When you're ready, do the same test again, but this time lift up the other leg.

One leg—the one with the tighter hip—should be MUCH more challenging to lift. This is the hip with the mobility restriction; it needs to get moving again. Meanwhile, the other hip (the looser one) probably feels very unsteady when you stand on it. This hip has a stability deficit—in other words, it isn't strong enough to support you, and so your body is compensating by putting most of its weight on the other side. The side with all the weight is being overworked and underpaid, which results in BACK PAIN!

How do you correct something like this? Simple: you strengthen the weaker hip!

Practice standing on one leg (yes, you have to stand on the leg that feels more unsteady—can't take the easy way out!) until you can hold the position for 60 seconds without using the counter. It will take a lot of time and effort, especially if you have been in pain for as long as Dolores was, but your body will thank you for it!

Skip ahead to the BONUS chapter at the end of this book for links to more absolutely free resources you can utilize to help you out with your back pain.

Chapter Nine:

Knee

· ·

Which do you think is more likely to break first: a sturdy piece of metal, or a wooden plank with holes drilled in it?

It's not a trick question—the answer is *definitely* the wood.

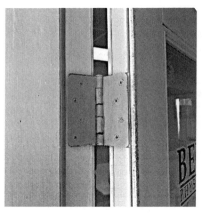

I'm talking about hinges. Your knee joint is considered a "hinge" joint. This is because it only moves back and forth, like a door hinge. Other joints are designed to twist and rotate, like your shoulders, or pivot, like your neck, but the knee only moves back and forth. Its job is to straighten and bend, and that's it.

Because of the simplicity of this joint, it's actually VERY easy to work on!

A number of clients who come to see me tell me their knee

pain is genetic: "My mom/dad had both knees replaced, so I'll have to have mine replaced, too." Others say they abused their knees early in life playing sports: "I played football back when we didn't use pads, and it just destroyed my knees." This type of explanation can be gratifying; it allows people to blame their pain on someone or something else.

Before we go any further, I want to be 100% clear that this chapter is strictly about non-traumatic knee pain. The knee pain we will be addressing does not have any specific "accident" that caused it—if you can trace the beginning of your pain back to one very specific tackle on the football field, your problem is considered "traumatic," because it originated due to a debilitating injury. If you have just lived your normal life and the knee pain just gradually set in over the years, then your pain is non-traumatic, and this chapter is going to speak directly to you.

So, why is the knee joint one of the easiest ones to work on?

Because the knee joint is rarely the actual problem!

The knee pain is a symptom of a different problem—and that problem is usually just above or below the knee joint. The most common cause of knee pain is hip dysfunction.

"But there's nothing wrong with my hips," you may be thinking—though I hope that by this point, you know better!

The Easiest Way To Fix Knee Pain Is By...Studying Doors?

Let's go back to the door hinge example. Think about the front door of your house. How often do you need to replace the hinges on that door?

Actually, scratch that.

Think about the front door of a Starbucks in New York City.

How many times does that door open and close every day? We can conservatively say it's in the thousands! People are in and out of Starbucks all day long, from the time it opens to the time it closes.

Have you EVER heard of someone needing to replace the hinges on a Starbucks door?

I haven't!

I've never heard of someone replacing the hinges on ANY door. Sure, if the hinge *breaks* because someone yanks open the door too hard (AKA, a traumatic event!), you'll need to get a new hinge. But hinges don't just "wear out" from overuse.

I'll give you an even MORE extreme example. My aunt lives in New England in a house that was built more than 100 years ago, in the early 1900s. Lots of maintenance has been done to that house over the years…but all of the original hinges are the same.

Now, my aunt HAS had some trouble in the past with her door frames starting to rot.

(Like we discussed earlier in the chapter, wood is going to break down MUCH faster than metal!)

When that happens, the screws in the hinges can start to get slightly looser as the wood in the door becomes weaker. Creaking noises may start now that the screws can't provide secure attachment to the door—the hinges have to strain to hold the up the weight of the door, because the door frame is too weak to provide enough support. But replacing the hinge will *never* fix the rotten wood of the door frame!

And getting a knee replacement will never solve the problems in your hips! Just like the rotting door frame can cause creaking and make you think you have defective hinges, a hidden dysfunction in your hip can cause pain in your knees and make you think you need a replacement.

Some people (and hopefully, you're not one of them anymore!) focus in on the hinges. They spray WD-40 to stop the noise; they replace the screws to give the hinges a firmer hold; they may even decide to buy new hinges altogether. But all of these things are temporary fixes, and the noise will keep coming back, because it's a *symptom* of a bigger problem with the door.

I can't stress this enough: it's not that the hinges are "wearing out" or that they're too weak to support the door. The problem is that *something else* is too weak to support *the hinges*!

The best solution, of course, is to replace the rotten wood of the door frame. Without a solid foundation, the screws will never stay in place tightly enough to hold onto the hinges, and the door will continue "hanging" by the hinges and causing that creaking.

Your Knees Are Collateral Damage

So let's unpack the metaphor: your knee joints are the hinges. Your hips and pelvis are the door and door frame—and the rot is a lack of stability and strength in those areas.

At the beginning of this chapter, I mentioned that the number one cause of knee pain is hip weakness. That's the rotten door frame—when the muscles in your hips are too weak, they stop supporting you the way they're supposed to, and you end up putting extra stress on your knees.

The most important muscle in the hip is the *gluteus medius.*

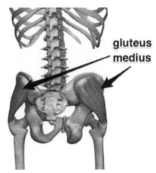

This muscle is used for walking, running, or any activity that requires you to stand on one leg. Weakness in this muscle causes the same instability as the rotting door frame! Without support from the door frame, the hinges have to work much harder than they were designed to work—and without support from the gluteus medius and the rest of the hips, the knees end up overworked, underpaid, and in pain!

Picture a supermodel doing that so-called "sexy walk."

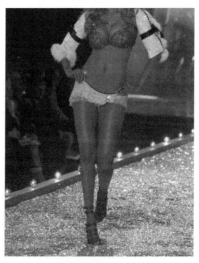

One of the model's hips is significantly higher than the other—which has thrown the rest of her body out of alignment!

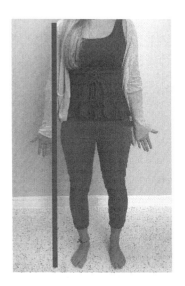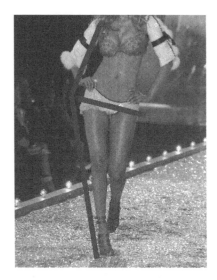

Tilting your hips and pelvis this far out of alignment puts an incredible amount of stress on the knee. Without your hip muscle there to support the weight of the top half of your body, the knee joint is forced to pick up the slack—and joints aren't designed to bear extra weight like that!

"But I don't walk like a runway model," you might be saying.

You're probably right! The runway model is a very extreme example, and on a scale of "correct walk" to "runway model walk," most people fall MUCH closer to the "correct" side. But even if you're 90% of the way to the "correct" walk, that last 10% will eventually take its toll! Door rot happens slowly, after all, but it *does* happen.

127

Doing This For Just 60 Seconds Per Day Can Significantly Reduce Your Knee Pain

So what can you do to correct your hip instability? There's no way to repair door frame rot, right?

Luckily, this is where our metaphor falls apart! It's completely possible to "repair" hip instability: all you have to do is strengthen those hip muscles. Once you can support your weight again, you won't need to rely on your knee joint to do the brunt of the work anymore, and it can go back to doing what it was designed to do in the first place.

Here's a very simple exercise you can do to strengthen the gluteus medius.

What we're going to do is practice keeping the pelvis level while standing on one leg.

Stand straight up with both feet side by side—they should be almost touching. Keeping both knees completely straight, pick up your left leg straight off the ground without letting your foot "swing" forward, backward, or sideways. You should only be able to pick your foot up an inch at the most!

You should begin to feel your right hip start to work after a few seconds. That's because this exercise is working on the right glute medius—if you were to stand on the other leg, you would feel the burn in the opposite hip.

Whichever side is more difficult to balance on is the side that needs strengthening. Usually, that side correlates to the side with the knee pain. It makes sense: the weaker hip is less stable and forces the knee to bear most of the weight, causing more pain!

Work on this exercise until you can hold both sides with perfect form for at least 60 seconds. The more you work, the less pain you should feel in your knees!

When The Hips Aren't The Problem

In some cases, knee pain is being caused by something *below* the knee: the foot!

In order to understand this, we need to talk about something called torsion.

Make a fist with both hands and touch your knuckles to each other, like you're giving yourself a "fist bump." The knuckles should be offset, so that they fit in between each other.

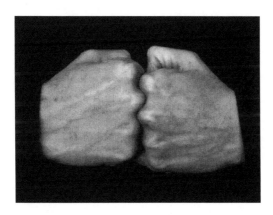

Experiment with which ways you can move your fists while they're in this position. You can probably slide them up and down relatively easily. But if you try to rotate one fist clockwise and the other counterclockwise, very minimal motion will occur. This motion is called *torsion*.

Your knee joint has a little bit of torsion, but not a lot. Imagine standing pigeon-toed, with both feet turned in toward each other; torsion makes that possible.

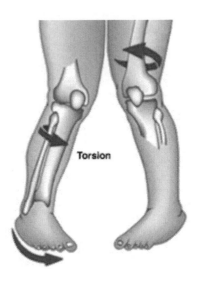

Twisting the knee too much will result in an injury (usually torn meniscus), but a little bit of twisting in a hinge joint is perfectly normal!

Let's go back to our door hinge example. Door hinges have torsion, too. It's so minimal that you would never be able to see it, but there is a slight torsion motion that occurs with every open and close. In a healthy door, you can only measure this twisting with advanced torque and force measurement equipment…but you can see it with the naked eye if you're looking at an "unhealthy" door!

Take that Starbucks door in New York City and picture a toddler hanging onto the handle and dangling as you open it. The toddler has superhuman strength; he hangs on all day, every day, for an entire week.

At first, it won't matter—the Starbucks door is built to withstand a lot of use, and the door will still open and close with ease. You won't hear any squeaking from the hinges. You won't have a problem with a rotten frame, since this door isn't 100 years old like my aunt's. The door will have doubled in weight with the toddler hanging on, but other than that, everything is normal.

As the week goes on, though, the hinges on that door are going to start feeling the effects of that extra weight. Each pound we add to the door increases the amount of work the hinges have to do— the hinges aren't getting worn out (they're metal! They don't "wear out!"), but they're not being used the way they were designed to be used, and they're going to start complaining about it.

By adding a toddler to the door, we have increased the amount of *torsion* in the hinges. Think about it: gravity is pulling the toddler toward the ground, and the toddler is dragging the door down with him. The door, in turn, will try to drag down the hinges —but the hinges are screwed firmly into the door frame, so they aren't going anywhere!

So now the hinges are being dragged in two directions: toward the ground, and toward the door frame. The result is a twisting motion—and the longer the heavy door pulls down on the hinge, the bigger that twist will become.

If you need a better way to visualize it, lock your fingers together in front of you. (Make sure your fists are facing away from you, so that if you give a "thumbs up," your thumbs point toward the ceiling.)

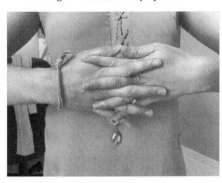

Try to pull one hand straight down toward the floor without moving the other hand. You shouldn't be able to do it; the interlocked fingers should make it impossible.

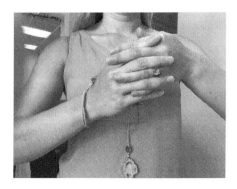

But the harder you try, the more your fingers should twist.

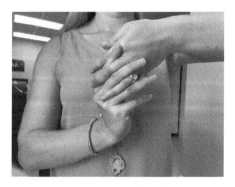

That's what's happening to our door hinges—they're twisting. It's a very, very small twist that you can't see with the naked eye, but the longer the door pulls on the hinge, the bigger the twist will become, until the door looks like this:

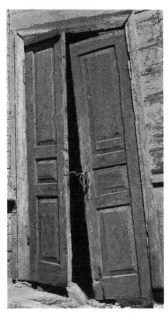

If we unpack this metaphor, we can see how our feet can cause knee pain. The hinge is, of course, your knee joint; the door is your foot; and the toddler hanging on the door is the *improper use of your foot.*

What does that mean?

It means that if your foot is not working the way it was built to work—for example, if you stand pigeon-toed, or if you walk with flat feet, or if you have any kind of limp—then you are applying extra torque to your knee and causing an increase in that torsion force. And, as you know, your knee wasn't built to handle a lot of torsion!

Just like the toddler hanging off the door, this foot problem won't show any signs immediately—it will take years, sometimes even decades, of improper walking/standing for your knee to start feeling the effects. But one thing is for sure: getting a knee replacement won't fix your foot, just like replacing door hinges won't change the weight of the toddler. The knee pain is a symptom of a much larger problem.

If you aren't sure whether your knee pain is coming from your hip or your ankle, consult a physical therapist! Skip ahead to the BONUS chapter at the end of this book for links to more absolutely free resources you can utilize to help you out with your knee pain.

Chapter Ten:

Foot

· ·

As I write this chapter, I'm sitting in the Atlanta airport, waiting for my flight home after a business trip, and I can't stop looking at everyone's shoes.

It started twenty minutes ago, when I saw a young woman running at full-speed through the airport to make it to her connecting flight…and she was wearing stiletto heels.

(I think. I'm no shoe expert.)

Now, first of all, I've never seen someone move so fast in high heels, so I was very impressed that she didn't fall on her face.

But it also got me thinking about how *horrendously bad* high heels are for your feet.

Was this woman an anomaly? Or was EVERY female in this airport wearing heels?

I looked around at the hundreds of people rushing past me, and I started to count.

During my hour-long layover, I saw just about every kind of footwear there is: tennis shoes, work shoes, dress shoes, flip-flops, wedges, lace-up sandals that go all the way to the knees, boots, crocs, light-up sneakers on kids, and high heel after high heel after high heel.

Somewhere during that period, I stopped paying attention to shoes and started noticing gait patterns. It's amazing how many people are unaware of what their walk looks like—a client of mine once came in for his initial appointment and seemed shocked when I told him he had a horrible limp!

But the truth is, most foot problems (and other problems, too!) are YEARS in the making. All the women running past in their heels had no idea what kind of damage they were doing to their feet—they were either used to the pain, really good at ignoring the pain, or convinced that the pain would go away when the shoes came off.

And it's true, when you're young. But as you age, the body becomes a less efficient healer, and all of the damage from wearing the wrong kind of shoe will start to catch up!

The foot is extremely complicated. It has over 100 tendons, ligaments, and muscles, as well as 26 bones and 33 joints—and they all work together to keep the foot stable and mobile. Taking a step requires perfect synchronization from every part of the foot, and if even one part stops working, your gait will suffer, creating a limp.

So when you take that perfectly orchestrated machine (your foot), and you shove it into a tight container that restricts its motion (AKA, a shoe!), you wind up with complications in your feet! With a shoe surrounding the foot, a lot of the muscles and joints no longer need to work. If your shoe has arch support, for example, your foot no longer needs to use its built-in "arch support" muscles—and so it just stops using them! Over time, your brain will literally forget how to engage these muscles, and so they will waste away and atrophy…which means that when you take off the arch-supporting shoes and put on flip-flops for the beach, your feet have no way to help support you, and you'll experience limping, instability, and pain.

The same principle applies if you're wearing heels every day: the tight restriction prevents certain parts of the foot from moving freely, and if you don't move 'em, you lose 'em!

Why Supportive Shoes Are The Wrong Answer—And Actually Make Things Worse

Foot pain usually starts because something about your routine changed.

Maybe you wore a different pair of shoes. Maybe you stood longer than you normally do at a holiday party. Maybe you visited NYC and walked more than you're used to walking.

(These are all real examples from people I've treated for foot pain!)

All of these examples involve increased stress on the foot, which is not trained to stand or walk anymore. The foot is just trained to do nothing. Its only job is to sit in a tight shoe.

When people first discover they have foot pain, the first thing they try is to buy a more comfortable shoe. This is the absolute *worst* route you can take! Now you're not only wearing a shoe that confines your foot and allows it to be lazy, but you're also adding a cushion to the bottom, which further decreases your brain's ability to perceive the foot!

What do I mean by that?

Stand on the floor right now and balance on one leg.

Now put a pillow on the floor and try balancing on one leg while standing on that.

The pillow makes everything more wobbly and less stable... which is exactly what a "comfortable" shoe will do for your foot. It makes the foot—which is literally designed to help you stay stable —*less stable!*

The only thing worse than a "comfortable" shoe is a "supportive" shoe, or an orthotic. An orthotic is a shoe insert designed to support the arch of your foot—and we already know that that kind of support causes muscles to atrophy!

"But I was born with flat feet!" you might be thinking. "This doesn't apply to me. I NEED the support."

I LOVE hearing this excuse!

Listen: just because you've always had flat feet doesn't mean you were born with different muscles. Everyone, from "high arch" people to "neutral foot" people to "flat feet" people, has the same muscles, tendons, ligaments, and bones in their feet.

The people with arch abnormalities are usually people who have worn shoes their entire lives. When we're infants, our parents put us in shoes—despite the fact we can't even stand up yet—just because the shoes are "cute." As we enter a crucial stage of physical development with our feet confined within shoes, we have no chance for proper growth! The shoes become a habit; the supportive muscles realize that they aren't needed, and they "retire" and atrophy. Because of that, the shoes become a *necessity*. We go to daycare and wear them all day. We rarely go outside without them. We aren't allowed to go to school without them. We aren't allowed to go to work without them (unless you work at Berman Physical Therapy!). Even at home, we sometimes wear slippers because the floor is just too hard on our poor, weak feet.

Your Brain Can Do This One Terrifying Thing In Less Than An Hour

Here's a little more insight on the connection between the brain and the muscles.

I remember reading about an EMG study while I was in PT school. (An EMG is a technique for evaluating and recording the electrical activity produced by skeletal muscles. Basically, it's a way to see which parts of your brain "light up" when you move certain muscles.)

The subject of the study was asked to wiggle the fingers on his right hand. Five areas of the brain lit up on the screen, each area correlating to one finger. Then they put the subject's hand in a three-fingered glove. The glove left his thumb and index fingers free, but it bound his middle finger, ring finger, and pinky together.

Here's an example of this kind of glove (although the one in the study wasn't a ski glove!).

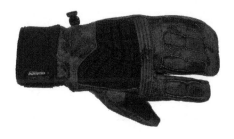

It only took 45 minutes for those five areas of the brain to blend together into three areas. Even though the subject was still wiggling all of his fingers individually, the brain had decided that the middle/ring/pinky fingers were all working as a single unit, and it changed its behavior accordingly.

When the glove came off, it took ANOTHER 45 minutes for the brain to differentiate between the five fingers again!

Dramatic changes in the brain can occur after keeping your hand stuck in a glove for only 45 minutes…so imagine what happens if you keep your feet stuck in shoes for *decades!*

Agnes Had Her Foot Pain "Under Control"…But She Was Actually Suffering Every Day!

A perfect example of how "support" can make foot pain worse is Agnes. Agnes is a 77-year-old client of mine who has lived in Naples for over 20 years now. She originally came to see me for low back pain, but as we worked together, I noticed that she had orthotics in her shoes.

"How long have you worn orthotics?" I asked her during one of our sessions.

Agnes told me she'd "needed" her custom orthotics for at least 40 years. "I can't take more than 20 steps without them," she said. "But they help a lot."

I asked if we could take a break from treating her back to focus on her feet. She initially refused—she and her orthotics had the foot pain "under control," she said.

"Under control?" I repeated. "You can't take 20 steps without being in pain! What happens in the middle of the night if you need a glass of water? How do you go to the beach or the pool with your grandchildren?"

Agnes thought about it. "I guess I'm limited," she said.

"Let's take a look at the feet," I said. "I think it might help fix the back pain, too."

I walked Agnes through a few balance tests to check the mobility of her feet. I asked her to stand on one leg, letting her use her fingertips for balance.

As I watched her try to remain stable, I noticed that she had her foot planted solidly on the floor, but she was still wobbling—she was trying to balance by moving her hips and shoulders into alignment over her foot, instead of using her foot muscles to support herself! She had gone for so long without using the stabilizing muscles in her feet that her brain had literally forgotten how to use them.

I gave Agnes three strengthening exercises to help her "wake up" the foot muscles she had forgotten how to use. It took seven weeks to undo 40 years' worth of damage, but by the end of her treatment, Agnes could stand on her right leg for 9 seconds and her left leg for 12 seconds—without holding on to anything, and without any wobbling! Her foot muscles finally learned to contract and relax to contribute to her balance.

Here's the really amazing part: now that Agnes could use the muscles in her foot, she was able to wean herself off the orthotics.

As soon as she did that, her back pain improved—not because the orthotics were directly hurting her back, but because they had been causing her to limp very slightly, which was throwing her back out of alignment!

Agnes ended up being discharged from my care *ahead of schedule!*

About eight weeks later, she called me up to brag about how she no longer wore shoes while working around the house or in the yard. "My feet haven't felt this good in...ever!" she told me. "I literally can't remember a time when they felt this good."

Imagine that: her feet felt better at age 77 than they had at *any other point in her life.*

"What are you going to do with those new feet?" I asked.

Agnes told me she wanted to travel to places she had always wanted to visit, but hadn't been able to because it required too much walking.

"San Francisco is the first place I want to go," she said. "I'm ready to make the dream a reality."

Let that sink in.

All it took to make her dream a reality was a few simple exercises to wake up the muscles in her feet—feet that she supposedly had "under control!"

How much do you think Agnes spent on custom orthotics and supportive shoes over her life? I asked her that very question, and she estimated that the answer was somewhere in the range of $10,000 to $15,000.

What would you do with an extra $15,000 in your bank account!? What would you take that trip that you've been talking about for 20 years? Would you invest it? Would you open up a college fund for your grandkid?

If it were me, I can guarantee you I wouldn't want to spend it on orthotics!

The Awful Truth About Orthotics

As we touched on briefly before, orthotics are shoe inserts that provide external support to the feet. We already know that external support is bad, and that it allows foot muscles to become lazy and eventually atrophy...so WHY are so many people recommending them?

The key is in the word "support." Support is a good thing—and we need it—but when it comes from something external, like orthotics, we end up relying on it in order to function normally. Like a caffeine addict needs a cup of coffee in the morning in order to prevent a headache, orthotics-wearers require their special inserts to walk without pain. And the longer you wear the orthotics, the more dependent you become, until even walking barefoot from your bedroom to the bathroom becomes unbearable, and you decide to pay a visit to your doctor or surgeon.

You know what would be great?

Internal orthotics! A support system that you never had to take off, that could never let you down or wear out, and that didn't cost a dime to maintain.

(By the way, you were born with all that—your feet muscles!)

Growing up, my grandparents had a house in Jamaica. The house was located up the mountain from Ocho Rios, close to an area called Fern Gully. It was a beautiful property overlooking the ocean, and I got to visit multiple times per year.

If you've ever been to Jamaica, or any Caribbean island, and have gotten away from the tourist-y part, then you know it's common to see people running around barefoot. The same is true in third-world countries across the globe—shoes really are a luxury item!

The same foot variations that we have here in America (pronated, supinated, and neutral) can be found in these third-world countries...but nobody there complains of foot pain!

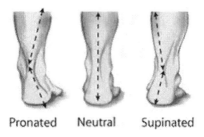

Pronated   Neutral   Supinated

When I was in Jamaica recently, I found myself looking at the locals' feet—just like I still am at the Atlanta airport right now! I saw all three types of feet, yet nobody was limping around. Nobody had any gait deviations. And everybody was barefoot!

How can all these Jamaicans walk around with pronated "flat" feet without wearing orthotics? And how can they do it without pain?

It's because most Jamaicans didn't grow up with shoes restricting their feet! They got the chance to grow, develop, and strengthen their feet without confining them to a tight shoe—which means that they have built-in support systems that will never compare to the external orthotics you can buy for hundreds of dollars.

So what's the solution to your foot pain?

Take your shoes off!

Don't quit cold-turkey—you've been wearing shoes all your life, and you'll end up in more pain if you take away the external support system without training the internal one, first. Walk around barefoot at home for half an hour a day, then work yourself up to an hour, then two hours, then more!

Another good exercise to try is a Towel Curl. Throw a bath towel on the floor, put your foot on top of it, and try to scrunch it up just using your toes. This will help wake up the intrinsic muscles in your foot, which means you're off to an excellent start!

If you're ready for your foot pain to be a thing of the past, a physical therapist could be your answer! Skip ahead to the BONUS chapter at the end of this book for links to more absolutely free resources you can utilize to help you out with your foot pain.

Bonus:

Your Health Resource Library

. . . .

You are now officially armed with all the knowledge you need to start treating your problems, not your symptoms. I hope you learned a lot, and, more importantly, had a great time!

If you would like more in-depth information and self-help tips on any of the common topics you see listed below, please visit the web address printed next to each. When you get there, you'll see a special tips report I created especially for you, and more information on ways to get the help you need.

Back Pain: www.bermanpt.com/back-pain/

Neck/Shoulder Pain: www.bermanpt.com/neck-shoulder-pain/

Knee Pain: www.bermanpt.com/knee-pain/

Please note that if any of the links should fail or change over time, you can ALWAYS navigate to the reports via our clinic's official website: www.BermanPT.com

You can also call our office at (239) 431-0232 to request a copy of one of our reports. Our selection is always growing.

Our most popular reports are:

- The Seven Most Common Causes of Neck&Shoulder Pain
- Your Complete Guide To Knee Pain
- Five Simple Ways to Prevent Another Fall
- The 20 FAQs of Physical Therapy
- The Six Most Common Causes of Back Pain
- 6 Questions to Ask Your Physical Therapist

If you would like to speak to a specialist about any health-related problem you're currently having, then I can also offer you a free 20-minute phone consultation with a physical therapist from my own clinic.

You can do that by visiting http://bermanpt.wpengine.com/telephone-consultation/ and filling in your information, or by calling my clinic directly at (239) 431-0232. Please tell the person answering the phone that you have been reading this book and wish to take advantage of the generous offer to speak with a specialist for free, and you will be taken care of.

Health Disclaimer

We make every effort to ensure that we accurately represent the injury advice and prognosis displayed throughout this book. However, examples of injuries and their prognosis are based on typical representations of those injuries that we commonly see in our physical therapy clinic. The information given is not intended to apply to every individual's potential injury. As with any injury, each person's symptoms can also vary depending upon background, genetics, previous medical history, application of exercise, posture, motivation to follow physical therapy advice, and various other physical factors.

It is impossible to give a 100% complete accurate diagnosis and prognosis without a thorough physical examination, and likewise the advice given for management of an injury cannot be deemed fully accurate in the absence of this examination from one of the physical therapists at Berman Physical Therapy.

We are able to offer you this service at a standard charge. Significant injury risk is possible if you do not follow due diligence and seek suitable professional advice about your injury. No guarantees of specific results are expressly made or implied in this book.